THE BEGINNERS GUIDE TO GROWING HERBS AND THEIR CULINARY, MEDICINAL, AND MYSTICAL PROPERTIES

By

GARY CARTER

THE BEGINNERS GUIDE TO GROWING HERBS AND THEIR CULINARY, MEDICINAL, AND MYSTICAL PROPERTIES
Copyright©2019 Gary Carter
All Rights Reserved
Published by Unsolicited Press
Printed in the United States of America.
First Edition 2019.

All rights reserved. Printed in the United States of America. No part of this book may be used or reproduced in any manner whatsoever without written permission except in the case of brief quotations embodied in critical articles or reviews.

Attention schools and businesses: for discounted copies on large orders, please contact the publisher directly.

For information contact:
Unsolicited Press
Portland, Oregon
www.unsolicitedpress.com
orders@unsolicitedpress.com
619-354-8005

Cover Design: Kathryn Gerhardt
Editor: S.R Stewart

ISBN: 978-1-950730-00-1

To my daughter Kimberly,

For her help in writing and editing this book and the two years it took to produce it.

Acknowledgements

I am grateful to my family and friends, and to those people in Port Orford, Oregon, whose encouragement and comments on my poetry and novels inspire me to keep writing. A special thanks to my daughter Kimberly James for her help in formatting, editing, and writing this book, and to my son Richard, without whose support this work would never have been conceived, written, or published.

Introduction

This book was conceived in a rather odd way, and for two different reasons. The first reason is, having been a plant grower off and on for some 30 years now, I never paid much attention to herbs. Probably because I have never had the time, or inclination, to learn how to be a gourmet cook. I grew some varieties, but they were plants like Rosemary and Thyme and things you could plant around the yard as ornamentals. However, moving to Curry County here on the southwestern Oregon coast presented a unique set of problems. One was the small population (23,000), along with a lack of new homes and businesses that generally buy the larger plants for landscaping purposes. My wife and I moved to Port Orford and had been retired from our tree-farm nursery business (in Tollhouse, California, in the foothills east of Fresno) for some time when she became ill and passed away from cancer in 2004. It was an expensive process and exhausted the small savings we had accumulated over the years. What to do? I don't have many skills outside of the plant business, so I started another nursery here at my home, only this time it was different. Going along with the switch by more people growing their own food and spices, I began growing herbs and vegetables along with some ornamentals, to sell at my home and at our local Farmer's Markets. Along with plants that grew well in our climate, and with a slew of vegetable choices, I grew a variety of herbs. I take pride in the fact that I can grow almost anything, anywhere, but I soon found out that I needed to know a lot more about the herbs I grew other than just how to plant them and keep them going. My early conversations at the Farmer's Markets went something like this:

"Pardon me sir, but do you grow any herbs?" the lady asked.

"I do. I have over twenty varieties of herbs with me today."

"Oh, good. Do you have cilantro?"

"I do," I answered, proudly pointing them out in my arrangement of herbs.

"Swell. What do you cook with them?"

"I'm sorry?"

"What does cilantro go good with? How do people use it? I'm starting an herb garden, and I need to know some things about what I buy before I decide."

"I'm sorry, mam, I'm not a cook. I just grow the things."

"Humph. Seems to me if you're going to grow herbs for people you should know something about them. I don't want to get poisoned!"

"Yes, mam," I answered as I watched her turn and walk away in a huff. This happened so many times my first year at the Farmer's Markets that I decided I was going to have to learn all about each and every herb if I was ever going to be successful at selling them. With that in mind I decided to write a book about the most common and most popular ones. Why not try and make a buck while you are learning?

The second reason I decided on this way of presenting herbs is that every herb book I researched, and all the websites I visited, wrote many, many pages on the herbs they had selected. While the content was interesting, it was much more than I had time to study or needed to know to find out about herbs. That is what prompted the idea on this scaled down version. There are books written solely on the culinary merits of herbs, on their medicinal values, and even on their mystical properties. I guess you could call this book a "Starter Book" for those wishing to get into the world of herbs. Along with a copy of a Sunset Garden Book for your area, the reference page toward the back of this book will show the reader where he, or she, may find books and websites much more detailed than they will find here, and your local library is always a good source. With these two thoughts in mind, I embarked on this adventure. It has been a grand and glorious ride. Not only have I found that herbs are culinary delights, but they have a myriad of alleged medicinal properties as well. Fact is, they have helped promote the wellness and health of humans down through the ages and in many cases dating back thousands of years. Most amazing to me on this journey, however, is that the vast majority of herbs carry magic with them, protecting you, your family and friends, your home, your business and just about everything else you value from evil, harm, spells cast upon you by others, and yes, even dragons. They also promote well-being, health, love, friendship and all the good things in life. I hope that you, the reader, will find as much joy and learning in reading, and using, this book as I did in researching and writing it.

Thank you!

Gary Carter

Table of Contents

	1
What Is An Herb?	15
Why Grow Herbs?	16
Organic Or Inorganic?	17
Disclaimer	19
A Short History Of Chinese Herbal Remedies	20
A Short History Of European Herbal Remedies	22
A Short History Of Middle Eastern Herbal Remedies	24
A Short History Of Eastern Indian Herbal Remedies	25
A Short History Of Native American Herbal Remedies	26
A Summary Of Herbal Remedies Through The Ages	27
Herbs	29
Aloe Vera	30
Angelica	32
Anise	34
Anise (Hyssop, Wonder Honey Plant)	36
Arugula	38
Australian Mint Bush	40
Basil	42
Bay Laurel (Sweet Bay)	44
Bee Balm (Bergamot, Oswego Tea, Horsemint)	46
Borage	48
Calendula (Pot Marigold)	50
Caraway	52

Catnip	54
Cayenne Pepper	56
Chamomile, German	58
Chervil (French Parsley)	60
Chicory	62
Cherry – Wild Black	64
Chickweed	66
Chives	68
Cilantro (Coriander)	70
Coneflower (Echinaceae)	72
Dandelion	74
Dill	76
Evening Primrose	78
Fennel	80
Feverfew	82
Garlic	84
Ginkgo (Maidenhair Tree)	86
Ginseng, American	88
Goldenrod	90
Goldenseal	92
Horehound	94
Hyssop	96
Lavender, English	98
Lemon Balm	100
Lemon Grass	102
Marijuana	104
Marjoram	106
Mint	108
Oregano	110

Parsley	112
Plantain (Ribwort)	114
Rosemary	116
Sage – Culinary	118
Saint John's Wort	120
Savory – Summer	122
Savory – Winter	124
Self-Heal (All-Heal)	126
Tarragon, French	128
Tarragon, Mexican	130
Thyme	132
Valerian (Garden Heliotrope)	134
Violet	136
Yarrow	138
An Introduction To Native American Herbs	141
An Introduction To Native American Herbal Remedies	142
Aspen – Quaking	144
Blackberry, American	146
Bladderpod (Fendler's)	148
Bloodroot	150
Blue Cohosh	152
Boneset (Feverwort)	154
Broom Snakeweed	156
Buckwheat, Red	158
Chokecherry	160
Creosote Bush	162
Devil's Claw	164
Dogbane (Indian Hemp)	166
Dogwood, Eastern	168

Evening Primrose (Sun Drop)	170
Geranium, Wild (Alum, Cransebill)	172
Honeysuckle (Trumpet)	174
Hops	176
Indian Paintbrush (Prarie Fire)	178
Lettuce, Wild (Canada Lettuce)	180
Licorice (Wild), American	182
Milkweed, Common (Butterfly Flower)	184
Mullein, Common	186
Oak, White	188
Partridge Berry	190
Pennyroyal, Eastern American	192
Pennyroyal, Western American	194
Persimmon, American (Sugar Plum)	196
Pokeweed, American	198
Queen Anne's Lace (Wild Carrot)	200
Red Raspberry, American	202
Sage – Antelope	204
Saltbush (Cattle Saltbush)	206
Sarsaparilla, Wild	208
Skunk Cabbage, Eastern Us	210
Skunk Cabbage, Western Us	212
Stargrass (Unicorn Root, Colic Root)	214
Stoneseed, Western	216
Sumac – Smooth Upland	218
Tobacco	220
Western Hemlock	222
White Pine, Eastern	224
Wild Onion (Garlic)	226

Willow, North American	228
Witch Hazel	230
Yellow Root	232
Yellow Spine Thistle	234
Bee Friendly Plants	237
Deer-Resistant Plants	245
How To Dry Herbs	249
How To Make Herbal Teas	250
How To Make Herbal Capsules	251
How To Make Herbal Oils And Ointments	252
How To Make Herbal Sodas	253
How To Make Herbal Candy	254
How To Make Herbal Incense	255
How To Make Herbal Candles	256
How To Make An Herbal Infusion, Decoction, Paste And/Or Poultice	257
Making An Herbal Poultice	259
Aromatherapy	260
Poisonous Plants	261
Human Ailments And Their Herbal Remedies	262
Native American Herbal Remedies	271
Zone Map	276
Glossary	277
References	279
About The Author	285
Also By Gary Carter	286

What Is an Herb?

There are more definitions of what an herb is than you can put in a book that one hand will hold. I like this one the best:

"Any plant that is used for its culinary, medicinal, aromatic or magical properties."

Humans have used herbs for thousands of years. As such, there are thousands of plants listed as herbs depending upon who you talk to or what resources you research. For this book, I have used what are considered the most common and useful herbs by historians, herbalists, gardeners, and nurseries alike, and have been the most used and categorized, down through the centuries. The reader will find that most herbs in mankind's history originated in Europe, Asia and the Middle-East. This is because on the African, Australian, North American, and South American continents there is no written history of herbs used by the indigenous people of those areas. That is not to say they didn't use them, there just isn't knowledge of them other than what has been handed down from "mouth to mouth" over the years, which is very little compared to other continents. As more people study herbs, many new, wonderful, and useful plants are popping up on these continents. The best is yet to come!

Like fruits, vegetables, and people, herbs come in all sizes, shapes, and colors. From groundcovers to bushes to trees. From annuals to perennials to biennials. Some smell good and some not so good. Some are invasive and some are not. There are those that prefer arid conditions and those that prefer moist. As you will see, however, most all of them are easy to grow, hardy and attract our friends the birds, bees, and butterflies, as well as, for some of them, deer. Not to worry, a table of "Deer Resistant Plants" is located toward the end of this book.

Why Grow Herbs?

Why grow anything? Most herbs not only provide us with beautiful flowers, but they attract some of our favorite friends: the birds, the bees, and the butterflies. Without them, we would have a difficult time surviving on this planet. As an added benefit, herbs provide seasoning for our food and many carry the added benefit of being medicinal. When I was a botany student at San Diego State back in the 1970's, I was researching a paper on some of the world's more famous plant people. Shortly after research began, it became apparent that people who deal with plants, whether exploring, gardening, farming or as nursery folks, on average live longer than people in any other profession. The reasons for this are self-evident: plant people work outdoors in fresh air and gardening provides a good source of all-around exercise as well as peace of mind. Not only that, growing your own herbs will add spice to your food, medicine to your cabinet, strength to your body, love to your heart and magic to your day.

What more can you ask?

Organic or Inorganic?

What's the difference?

One of the most confusing aspects of gardening to the beginner is the terms "organic" and "inorganic." What's the difference? Organic compounds contain the element carbon, and inorganic do not. Compost is a good example of the former, and fertilizers such as 16-16-16 and Miracle Gro the latter. Plants, however, do not know the difference. In the garden they will take up the necessary "ions" for their growth regardless of what kind of fertilizer is applied to the soil. Specifically, plants do not need soil, or compost either, to grow well. Hydroponic (soil-less) farming proves this point. Why all the fuss about "going green" and not using inorganics in your garden? This is addressed below.

Hydroponics aside, compost and natural manures keep your soil healthy in many ways that inorganics cannot. They build soil stability, provide a home for soil organisms beneficial to your plants, improve tilth, hold moisture, and absorb carbon, helping to reduce mankind's "carbon footprint" and climate change on our planet. Eventually, without the reapplication of organics into your soil on a regular basis, your garden will break down and be unable to support healthy plant and animal life, resulting in erosion, wind damage, etc. to the soil.

But composts and manures are impractical for large gardens and container gardening. In my nursery, to go around and apply a handful of steer manure, or compost, to roughly 10,000 plants, on a regular basis, is highly inconvenient, expensive labor wise and impossible to achieve economically. The same holds true for large nurseries and farms, and, unless you have a lot of time on your hands, impractical for the home gardener too. What to do?

While a botany student at San Diego State, I devised an experiment to try and settle this dispute, as least to my personal satisfaction. I mixed some soil from my yard half-and-half with compost and put this mixture into 12 separate 8" clay pots. I planted zonal geraniums in three pots, lettuce in three pots, petunias in three pots, and onion in three pots. On the soil surface of the first group of four pots (1 geranium, 1 lettuce, 1 petunia and one onion bulb), I applied a handful of steer manure once a month. Into the second set of pots (same mix of plants), steer plus a teaspoon of 16-16-16, and into the third set only a teaspoon of 16-16-16. Over a period of three months, the plants fertilized with manure did okay, but did not grow very fast or flower very well. The second group flourished, and the last group did well for a while and then went into decline. My conclusion is a mixture of both inorganic and organic materials in your garden gives the best overall effect, and that is the formula I have stuck to in my yard, garden and nursery over the years which has proven highly effective. Recently, however, due to the rising demand for organic fruits and vegetables, I have taken to using strictly blood and bone meal on my herbs and vegetables. While the plants don't grow as fast overall as the organic-inorganic mixtures, they do very well otherwise and, according to recent research, are healthier for you.

Inorganics have their place. If your tomato plant looks healthy, but is not producing flowers and fruit, some 'super bloom' should help, giving you the desired results quicker than repeated applications of organic materials. If your hedge is not growing fast enough to suit you, some Miracle Gro to go along with your organics should get them moving. Nowadays, when you buy "organic" produce, the term simply means the products you are buying have not been sprayed with any harmful pesticide or fungicide. It used to be the term included plants grown using organic composts, manures and the like but, for a while now, the USDA has abandoned the term in regard to fertilizers. In sum, the term "organic," as applied to vegetables and fruits, has nothing to do with the fertilizer, or soil, used to help them grow.

One of the biggest drawbacks to using inorganic fertilizers is that, besides destroying your soil and its beneficial organisms over time, excess material will leach into the ecosystems that surround your garden, including waterways, with serious consequences. Excess manures have the same effect, leaching nitrogen and other elements into waterways, promoting algae and other undesirables, eventually destroying the ecological balances there. Always use the recommended amounts of fertilizers, both organic and inorganic, when gardening as too much, or too little, of either will not produce the desired effects.

This is a contentious issue. Proponents on opposite sides of the fence can almost come to blows telling one side or the other that their methods are best. Rest assured there is no known case of anyone dying or getting leprosy because they did not use organic fertilizers in their garden, nor has any cow died in a pasture for the same reason. If interested, Google "organic vs. inorganic" and spend your next three weeks reading up on the pros and cons. As for me, my little experiment has served me well over the 45 or so years that I have been a plant grower and gardener.

Disclaimer

WARNING!

Always be careful when using herbs in any capacity. They can be harmful if used in the wrong manner or in the wrong quantities. Consult your doctor, an herbalist, a chef, or a reliable cook if you are in doubt about any aspects of what you are doing, or planning to do, while using herbs. Consult the internet on the herbs of your choice and read what information is available. It is generally advised that pregnant women not use herbs during their pregnancy, especially for medicinal purposes. Make sure the plant you are using is the correct plant. Plants bought in stores can, and have been, mislabeled. If you are uncertain, visit your local nursery, garden club or any other plant professional for help with plant identification. Gathering wild herbs, whether from roadsides or other places, is considered inadvisable due to possible spraying of poisonous insecticides and herbicides by road crews, farmers, and the like. The reader of this book assumes all risks associated with the use of any material in this book.

To ease your mind, members of my family, many of my friends, acquaintances and their families, and their friends and acquaintances, have been cooking with herbs for culinary and medicinal purposes for as long as I can remember. While no one has ever become ill or died from using herbs that I know of, make sure you have done the proper research before using your plants.

That said, let's get started!

A Short History of Chinese Herbal Remedies

The Chinese and Asian Continents have had a long history of herbal remedies. Perhaps even the longest in the history of mankind. Not only did they use plants in their repertoire, they included animal parts along with chemical and biological substances. Chinese history states that a person named Shennong started experimenting with herbs, did okay for a while, then was poisoned. Indeed, how did one go about finding out which plants were poisonous, and which were not, in ancient times? I envision some person, along with his/her family, who were starving, out combing the countryside, and sampling this plant or that, hoping he/she would find one or more to eat that didn't make her/him sick or kill them. How else could they have done it? According to Native American folklore their people watched what wild animals ate in plant materials and harvested those same plants for their own usage. Who is to say the early Chinese didn't do the same? While this didn't always work, as some plants eaten by animals are poisonous to humans, it sounds like it was a good place to start. All things considered, it must have been a long, hard row to hoe for our ancient ancestors in learning the art of herbology.

The first traditionally recognized herbologist went by the name of "Shennong" (translated as "Divine Flower"). A Chinese, mystical god-like creature, he allegedly tasted hundreds of herbs and imparted his knowledge of medicinal plants to farmers. "*Shennong's materia medica*" is considered by most as the oldest book (2800 B.C) on Chinese herbal medicines. It classifies 365 species of roots, grass, woods, furs, and stones into three categories of herbal medicine.

Dating back from 2500 B.C. to around 2200 B.C. there is mention of alcohol and soups as medicines. Also from around 1100 B.C. to 771 B.C. "The Book of Songs" was compiled that mentions information about medicines.

The earliest "true" book on Chinese herbal medicinal plants (basically translated from Chinese into "Roots and Shoots") was written from 221 B.C. to 220 A.D. and was based on the work of medical experts who collected plants and tested them for their value. This book recorded some 365 types of medicine, some of which are still being used today. The book is credited with putting the beginnings of eastern medicine into circulation.

One of the earliest lists of prescriptions for specific ailments, titled "*Recipes for 52 Ailments*", was found in the "Mawangdui" tombs, which had been sealed in 168 B.C. The list has expanded down through the centuries and, in 1977, a book titled "*Herbal*

Medicine Dictionary" (translated) contained some 5,767 herbal medicines. Today, there are roughly 13,000 medicines used in Chinese herbology and over 100,000 recipes recorded from ancient literature.

So, the next time you are in the market for some Chinese herbs, you might want to stop and thank all those older generations of Asian people who risked their lives in order that their brethren might live longer, happier, and healthier lives.

A Short History of European Herbal Remedies

The first known record of Europeans using herbs is credited by many people to the Greek physician Hippocrates (460-377 B.C.), putting Europeans well behind the Asian and Middle Eastern regions in developing these lines. Borrowing from the Egyptians and Mesopotamians he developed a system of diagnosis and prognosis using herbs. He considered illness a natural, not supernatural (like those before him) occurrence, and maintained that medicine should not be given in the same concert with superstition. In 77 A.D., Pliny the Elder wrote 37 volumes on natural history, devoting seven of them to the medicinal use of plants. Unfortunately, much of what Pliny wrote on this issue was never verified and of not much value today.

An ancient physician by the name of Galen (131-201, A.D.) developed a system called "humors", linking a person's body type to his health and personality. For the next 1400 years, physicians would trust in Galen's principals for better or for worse, often using his ideas for bizarre medical practices. One physician dared to break rank with "humors" in the 16th Century. A man named Paracelsus (1495–1541, A.D.) would argue that any botanical that bore a resemblance to human parts, if used, would heal those parts. Got a broken finger, eat a carrot. Good luck with those ideas!

The progress of science and the understanding of plants in Europe nearly collapsed with the fall of the Roman Empire. The early Middle Ages saw a return to the superstitions and rituals that surrounded herbs. Some herbs were given a bad name during this period. A common misconception was that scorpions bred beneath Basil grown in pots, and inhaling the Basil's scent, would drive scorpions into your brain. Because of its collapse, much of the learning by their predecessors was lost to the population at large. Despite this, many cultures in the Middle Ages possessed a sophisticated knowledge of medicinal herbs as evidenced by archaeological finds. Your average person during this era could still make use of local herbs to flavor foods and act as medicines. During this time, lords and other higher-ups began importing herbs, such as cinnamon and spice, from the Far East, giving rise to the belief that paradise existed somewhere "over there" as evidenced by the new and exciting plants being imported.

As Europe emerged from the Middle Ages, trade with other civilizations increased. In fact, the discovery of the new world was funded by a quest for new herbs and spices as witnessed by the explorations of Columbus, who was seeking new and less expensive trade routes to the Far East. During the Renaissance, nobles began filling their libraries with vast amounts of human knowledge, including herbs.

The first comprehensive herbal was published by Englishman Nicholas Culpepper in 1692. The physician systematically cataloged all the known herbal remedies of the time and dedicated his efforts to the common people. In essence, he showed them how they could rely on their own herbal remedies rather than the expensive concoctions of doctors. Needless to say, the physicians of his day were prone to dislike him. Herbalists tend to not be liked too much by today's doctors either, and for the same reason.

In the 18th Century, Swedish botanist Carl von Linné, better known as Linnaeus, developed the system of binomial nomenclature, which spearheaded a division between botany and herbalism. In early times, scholars discovered and examined plants with an eye on their usefulness in relation to human ailments. The Linnaean system placed a greater emphasis on cataloging plants without regard for usefulness. As a result, more information was lost using plants for medicinal and culinary purposes.

With that occurrence, western medicine would eventually disregard herbalism in favor of chemical cures. In some parts of the western world, herbology was actually outlawed when not practiced by a doctor with conventional medical training, and still is in some cases. Marijuana is a prime example.

With the advent of chemical medicines on the market, it was felt for a time that herbal medicine would no longer be necessary but that has not been the case. Chemical remedies for sickness are not "magic bullets" and in some cases cause more harm than good. With that herbal medicines are making a comeback, which is another reason for writing this book. Like Doctor Culpepper advocated, there can be better, cheaper ways to take care of yourself and avoid the horrendous costs of modern medicines.

A Short History of Middle Eastern Herbal Remedies

The earliest medical prescriptions involving plants come from ancient Mesopotamia around 5000 B.C., some 2200 years before recorded Asian medical recipes, and are written in Sumerian. They involved "medical professionals" and "magic dispensing individuals" working together to try and cure sick people.

Babylonian medical texts from the era prescribe a great many plant products, such as leaves, blossoms, seeds, and roots to be prepared and administered to the ill. Like their Asian counterparts, they also included animal parts and minerals in their arsenal.

Later, the search for cures from the natural world stemmed from the prophet Mohammed who taught that "God has provided a remedy for every illness."

Around 1500 B.C., the ancient Egyptians wrote the "Ebers Papyrus," which contains over 850 plant medicines.

During the 9th Century, a medical school using plants, known as "Bimaristan" (hospital), appeared among the Persians and Arabs, who were more advanced than their counterparts in Europe at the time. As a trading culture the Arab world had access to herbs from distant places such as India, China, and Africa. Muslim botanists and physicians significantly expanded on earlier knowledge of other medical professionals. For example, al-Dinawari described more than 637 plant medicines in the 9th Century. Ibn-al-Baitar described more than 1400 different plants, foods, and drugs during the 13th Century. The Andalusian-Arab botanist, Abu-al-Abbas-al-Nabati, introduced imperial techniques used in the testing, description, and identification of numerous "materia medica" (medical material/substance) and separated unverified reports from those supported by actual tests and observations. This allowed the study of *materia medica* to evolve into the modern science of pharmacology.

Baghdad was an important center of civilization between 800 A.D. and 1400 A.D., promoting, among other things, the advance of herbal medicine.

Most important is that the Middle Eastern countries, with their extensive network of east-west trade routes, expedited the spread of herbal knowledge regarding medicine, food, cosmetics, and fragrances around the world. Like the Chinese and Eastern Indians at the time, this knowledge helped ease, through ancient herbology, human suffering and pain and helped advance humanity under more comfortable conditions.

A Short History of Eastern Indian Herbal Remedies

Ayurveda, which stands for "Knowledge of Life" in India, mixes religion with secular medicine. Today, more than eighty percent of India's population relies on herbal remedies as the principle means of preventing and curing illness.

Ayurvedic medicine is a holistic system with great emphasis on prevention to help people live long, healthy, and well-balanced lives. Incorporating herbs in its teachings has been practiced in India for at least 5,000 years, and the concept of Ayurveda is considered by many scholars to be the oldest healing science on earth.

India was one of the first countries to focus on medicinal plants for healing. Today, there are approximately 1,400 plants used in Ayurvedic medicine.

The "Atharvaveda" is a sacred text of Hinduism. Written around 600 B.C., it is the first Eastern Indian text dealing with medicine based on the concepts concerning the exorcism of demons and magic. This text also contains prescriptions of herbs for various ailments. The use of herbs to treat ailments would later form a large part of Ayurveda.

Due to its complexity it is beyond the scope of this book to give a better picture of Eastern Indian medicinal and culinary uses of herbs, but there are hundreds of websites that will give a more detailed analysis of these ancient Indian practices to the interested person.

A Short History of Native American Herbal Remedies

According to Native American folklore, "The Creator," or "Great Spirit," supplied many ways to heal the body and for every human ailment there was a cure provided by Mother Nature. The typical tribal medicine man, or woman, was well equipped to treat a wide range of medical needs from the common cold to complications arising from childbirth. This required a vast knowledge of plants and plant cures passed down from generation to generation. In return for this service, the medicine man, or woman, was well cared for and protected by those in the village. In return, the medicine man, or woman, took care of the physical and emotional health of the tribe.

By the time European settlers arrived in America, there were over 2,000 Native American tribes fully established with sustainable medical procedures. As in other cultures, Native American medicine combined herbs, animal parts and minerals, along with spiritual rituals and magic, to cure the sick. Unfortunately, because of the early exploitation of Native Americans, along with no written records, many Native American herbal remedies have long been forgotten.

A Summary of Herbal Remedies Through the Ages

As long as 60,000 years ago, plants were associated with the spiritual side of mankind as shown by the discovery of a grave containing the remnants of a Neanderthal man in the Middle East who was buried with six different varieties of plants. Scholars hypothesize that the plants were put there to help the deceased get to some spiritual Nirvana believed to exist in that ancient time.

That aside, modern belief, as evidenced by records, has estimated that a general knowledge of herbal medicine existed as far back as 5,000 years ago and began with the Stone Age. Written records go back around 2,000 years in both Asia and Europe. The earliest significant Western documents on medicine are from ancient Egypt. From there, the knowledge of herbal medicines was passed on to the Greeks and the Romans. The knowledge of medicine subsequently flowered in Persia and the Middle East, then from Southern Europe at several schools in Italy around the 15th and 16th Centuries. The late 14th Century saw the invention of the printing press and the first two books to ever be printed were the Bible and a family herbal.

As far as America is concerned, the first settlers from Europe brought their herbal medicines and plants with them, some of which have now naturalized. The Europeans took the knowledge back, as well as many plants that Native Americans used, some of which have naturalized in Europe and the Middle East as well. It was during this time that trade between east and west was at a high point and the herbs of the world, and their healing powers, began spreading across the globe to the eventual betterment of all mankind.

From my own viewpoint, after much research, it is evident that there is a vast array of information on this subject. It would appear no two authors agree on exactly the what, when and where of herbal history. There is, however, an overall consensus about the dates, methods and circumstances concerning herbal history. Interestingly enough, those that espouse the virtues of early herbalism in Europe fail to mention that, at about the same time, the same discoveries and practical uses of herbs were also under way in China, and vice versa. Whatever the case, it appears that the knowledge and uses of herbs spread across the globe during an almost identical time frame and has continued into present day. Thankfully, many of the old misconceptions about herbs have been proven false, and the use of herbs as viable medicinal remedies are gathering strength, once again, as an alternative to pills, shots, operations, and the like.

Okay, enough preamble, let's look at some herbs and their uses. We'll start with Aloe Vera, perhaps one of the greatest medicinal plants to ever grace our planet.

Herbs

ALOE VERA

Aloe vera

Family	Asphodelaceae – Lily family
Origin	Africa
Zones	8, 9, 12-24, h1, h2; needs temperatures above 40° to grow properly
Type	Perennial
Inclination	Non-invasive
Exposure	Full to half-sun; indoors in a well-lighted window
Start	Leaves or seeds; cut at leaf base and let raw part dry before planting in clean sand; keep sand (or perlite) moist but not wet, and give good light and air circulation to prevent rot; seeds are slow to start
Growth	To 4' x 4'
Flowers	Yellow flowers in dense spikes, to 3' tall
Harvest	Anytime
Fertilizer	Liquid plant food
Soil	Well-drained
Tolerance	Keep on dry side; does not tolerate wet soil
Attracts	Bees
Seaside	Yes
Containers	Yes; indoors in cold weather (below 40°)

USES

CULINARY — While some websites advocate the usage of Aloe vera for drinking, eating, etc., as of this writing there are differing opinions on whether or not this plant is suitable to ingest. We highly recommend you see your doctor before consuming any Aloe products.

MEDICINAL — Cut leaves from plant and use juice to help heal insect bites, scratches and irritations, herpes, rashes, blisters, fungus, vaginal infections, conjunctivitis, sties, dry skin and allergic reactions, acne, sunburn, frostbite, shingles, psoriasis, rosacea, warts, wrinkles from aging and eczema. Internally (do not ingest leaves – buy pills, drinks, or jellies, etc.), Aloe Vera is professed to help treat congestion, indigestion, stomach ulcers, colitis, hemorrhoids, liver problems, kidney infections, urinary tract infections and prostate problems. The use of this plant in the industry is unregulated, so proceed with caution when using pills or other remedies. Always read the labels to make sure you are buying the right concoction for what ails you.

MYSTICAL — Leaves hung in doorways are said to attract luck and protect from evil influences. An Aloe Vera plant growing in the kitchen is thought to protect against accidents involving fire, burns or heat. A potted plant growing in the work place is supposed to bring good luck. Cleopatra is said to have used Aloe gel to preserve her beauty and the same can be said for Josephine, Napoleon's wife, who used a mixture of Aloe and milk. Over the centuries, Aloe Vera has been linked magically with beauty and healing. So, go for it!

ANGELICA

Angelica archangelica

Family	Apiaceae – Carrot or Parsley family
Origin	West Asia and northern Europe
Zones	A2, a3, 1-10, 14-24
Type	Perennial, biennial
Inclination	Non-invasive
Exposure	Half-sun
Start	Sow seeds directly into ground in spring, late summer or fall; Angelica has a taproot and does not transplant easily
Growth	To 3'x3'; flower stalks to 6' x 4'
Flowers	Yellow-green umbrella like clusters of flowers grow in early summer; keep stalks and flowers cut to prolong life; fragrant
Harvest	Roots in fall of first year; leaves in spring of second year; seeds when ripe
Fertilizer	Organic, all-purpose
Soil	Rich, well-drained
Tolerance	Always keep moist; deer resistant
Attracts	Bees
Seaside	Yes
Containers	Not recommended

USES

CULINARY — Angelica, from seeds to roots, imparts a licorice taste. The roots combine well in yeast breads, cakes, muffins, and cookies. The stems can be candied and/or used to decorate cakes and puddings. Fresh leaves can be used in salads, soups, stews and as a garnish. Roots and leaves are used to flavor liqueurs such as Benedictine and Chartreuse, and the roots are used to flavor gin and vermouth.

MEDICINAL — An infusion has been used for bronchial problems and as an expectorant. As a cough syrup boil 2-3 roots in a quart of water. Strain and add honey for consistency. Take 2 tablespoons up to 3 times a day for relief of coughs and congestion. A cup of homemade tea is professed to aid in digestion after meals and to help ease the pain of arthritis. Drink 1-2 cups a day. Add honey as a sweetener. Place some Angelica leaves in a cheesecloth bag, or some old hosiery, and drop in the tub for some homemade aromatherapy.

MYSTICAL — Myths and legends have surrounded Angelica for centuries. It is said to bloom every year on May 8, the feast day of the Archangel Michael, thus the name Angelica archangelica. Grow it in your garden to protect your home. Make leaf necklaces or carry the root in your pocket or purse for protection. Sprinkle in all corners of the house to ward off evil spirits or burn the dried leaves to impart a joyful outlook to those living in the house.

ANISE

Pimpinella anisum

Family	Apiaceae – Carrot or Parsley family
Origin	Asia and eastern Mediterranean
Zones	1-24 – h1, h2
Type	Annual
Inclination	Non-invasive
Exposure	Full-sun
Start	Seeds in spring but needs four months of growth for seeds to set; plant after all danger of frost is past and when ground has warmed up; anise has a tap root and does not transplant easily
Growth	To 2' x 1'
Flowers	Small clusters of tiny, white flowers at stem tips; fragrant
Harvest	Leaves and seeds
Fertilizer	Organic, all-purpose
Soil	Light, well-drained and slightly alkaline
Tolerance	Average water
Attracts	Bees, butterflies, and hummingbirds
Seaside	Yes; needs protection from strong winds
Containers	Yes

USES

CULINARY Anise seeds are used to flavor cakes, breads, eggs, fruit, and cheese. Fresh chopped leaves are appealing in soups, stews, sauces, and salads. Several liqueurs are made from the plant, as well as a refreshing tea. It is best to buy the whole seed (or use your own) and grind it yourself as needed. Already ground Anise quickly loses its flavor and aroma.

MEDICINAL Anise tea is used to cleanse the palate and settle the stomach after a heavy meal. The seeds are given to children to relieve colic and nausea and help in countering menstrual pain, asthma, bronchitis, and spasmodic coughs. Anise is also an effective expectorant and contains the compounds dianethole and photoanethole, which are similar to the female hormone estrogen, and has been recommended by traditional herbalists for nursing mothers and to help in relieving menopausal hot flashes. Three cups of tea a day are recommended. Anise is also used as an anti-flatulent and, externally, anise tea, soaked in a compress, can be used to help alleviate eye pain. Seeds mixed into a glass of warm milk, prior to bed time, are reputed to help insomnia and the seeds, when chewed in the morning, can act as an all-day mouth freshener.

MYSTICAL Burning the seeds has been used traditionally in protection and meditation incenses. Sleeping on a pillow stuffed with Anise seeds is supposed to prevent nightmares, and a sprig of anise hung on your bedpost will reputedly revive departed youth.

ANISE (HYSSOP, WONDER HONEY PLANT)

Agastache foeniculum

Family	Lamiaceae – Mint family
Origin	North America
Zones	A3, 1-24
Type	Herbaceous perennial
Inclination	Non-invasive; may reseed under proper conditions
Exposure	Full to half-sun
Start	Cuttings or divisions in late spring or early summer, seeds in early spring
Growth	To 2' x 3'
Flowers	Generally, dark blue on spikes; other shades available; fragrant
Harvest	Flowers, leaves (when young) and seeds
Fertilizer	Organic, all-purpose
Soil	Well-drained
Tolerance	Some drought resistance once established; deer resistant
Attracts	Bees, butterflies, hummingbirds, finches, and other wild birds
Seaside	Yes
Containers	Yes

USES

CULINARY — Anise leaves are delightful (dried or fresh) for tea or as a culinary seasoning. Licorice-mint smelling leaves and seeds can be used sparingly in salads, stews, and marinades, in poultry stuffing, soups, beverages and as flavoring in breads, cakes, and cookies

MEDICINAL — There are three plants classified as Anise; "Anise Hyssop" is the North American variety and, as such, unlike Europe and Asia, there is little history on the uses of this plant for medicinal purposes. However, Native Americans used the leaves in the treatment of chest pains from too much coughing, and a poultice of the leaves was used to treat burns.

MYSTICAL — The Cheyenne, and other Native North American tribes are said to have used the leaves for a "dispirited heart," probably as a tea. The Chippewa are said to have used the plant as a charm for protection.

ARUGULA

Eruca sativa

Family	Brassicaceae – Cabbage family
Origin	Mediterranean
Zones	All zones
Type	Annual
Inclination	Arugula is a cool weather plant; reseeds under proper conditions
Exposure	Full sun in cooler locations; ½ sun in hotter climates
Start	Seeds; plant in winter or early spring; successive plantings for year-round crops
Growth	To 2' x 1'
Flowers	Small, white, or yellow with crimson or violet veins and dark centers; fragrant
Harvest	Flowers and young leaves for salads; older leaves for cooked greens
Fertilizer	Organic
Soil	Well-drained
Tolerance	Average water; keep soil moist.
Attracts	Bees
Seaside	Yes
Containers	Yes

USES

CULINARY   Use young leaves for salads and stir-fry dishes. Older leaves can be cooked along with other greens. Leaves and flowers have a nutty taste and are a component of mesclun, a mixture of lettuces, chicories, endives, and other mild herbs.

MEDICINAL   High in vitamins A and C.

MYSTICAL   Arugula (also called Rocket Salad) usage dates to the first century, AD, where it was supposedly used as an aphrodisiac, and in Roman times the leaves and seeds were used for flavoring oils.

AUSTRALIAN MINT BUSH

Prostanthera rotundifolia

Family	Lamiaceae – Mint family
Origin	Australia
Zones	5, 14-17, 19-24
Type	Evergreen perennial
Inclination	Non-invasive
Exposure	Part-sun or shade; shade required in hotter climates
Start	Cuttings or seeds, plant spring or summer
Growth	To 8'x 5'
Flowers	Profuse purple-blue to rose-pink; leaves are fragrant
Harvest	Leaves
Fertilizer	Organic, all-purpose
Soil	Well-drained
Tolerance	Always keep moist
Attracts	Bees
Seaside	Yes; needs protection from wind
Containers	Yes

USES

CULINARY — Australian Mint Bush is just coming into its own in the culinary market and is a plant that needs more research; however, its leaves have been used as a substitute for thyme, have a strong mint smell and flavor, and can be used to make tea or flavor soups and salads.

MEDICINAL — Its leaves are antibacterial, antifungal, and carminative. The leaves can also be ground into a pulp and rubbed onto the chest, similar to Vicks, to help alleviate congestion. Boiled in water the fumes can be breathed to help clear the lungs, make breathing easier and to help with colds, headaches, and migraines.

MYSTICAL — Coming from Australia, there is not much history aligned with Mint Bush. What is known is that the Aborigines used it as an infusion for relief of headaches and colds.

BASIL

Ocimum basilicum

Family	Lamiaceae – Mint family
Origin	India
Zones	All zones
Type	Annual
Inclination	Non-invasive
Exposure	Full sun or indoors in well-lighted window
Start	Seeds in early spring; best results if set out after all danger of frost is past
Growth	To 2' x 2'
Flowers	White flowers on spikes; purple flowers on purple basil; fragrant
Harvest	New leaves best; pinch flower stalks to prolong season
Fertilizer	Time release or liquid; plants are sensitive, "hard" fertilizers will burn them
Soil	Rich, well-drained
Tolerance	Average water; keep on dry side to avoid stem rot; prefers warm soil; keep above 50° at all times
Attracts	Bees
Seaside	No
Containers	Yes; requires protection from wind

USES

CULINARY — Basil is one of the world's most widely used herbs. Its aromatic leaves are used to flavor soups, salads, fish, poultry, meat, spaghetti, pesto, etc. Basil has also been used to make a refreshing tea and as a garnish.

MEDICINAL — Basil, once made into a tea, is used for its digestive and anti-gas properties as well as being recommended for stomach cramps, vomiting, constipation, headaches, and anxiety.

MYSTICAL — To the ancient Greeks and Romans Basil was a symbol of malice and lunacy. In French, "semer le basilica" (sowing basil) means "ranting." In other cultures, the herb is associated with love rituals. In Eastern Europe, if a woman handed a man a sprig of Basil, and he accepted it, then that man would grow to love the woman. In Italy, when a woman placed a pot of Basil on her balcony it meant that she would be receptive to her lover. A plant near the doorway of your business, or a sprig in the cash register, is said to bring in more customers and to help you prosper. To protect your home and family, place Basil in all four corners of the house and replace monthly.

BAY LAUREL (SWEET BAY)

Laurus nobilis

Family	Lauraceae – Laurel family
Origin	Mediterranean
Zones	5-9, 12-24, h1, h2
Type	Evergreen small tree
Inclination	Non-invasive
Exposure	Full to half-sun
Start	Fresh, green cuttings or seeds; Bay Laurel is slow growing; therefore, it is recommended that they be purchased already well-rooted
Growth	To 12'- 40' and as wide
Flowers	Small, yellow flowers in spring followed by dark, purple-black berries; fragrant
Harvest	Leaves: anytime
Fertilizer	Organic, all-purpose
Soil	Well-drained
Tolerance	Average water; drought tolerant once established
Attracts	Bees and butterflies
Seaside	Yes
Containers	Yes

USES

CULINARY Use Bay Laurel leaves whole, then remove after cooking as leaf edges are sharp and can cut or stick in the throat. Bay Laurel can be used in any dish using a liquid. It is well known for flavoring soups, stews and tomato sauce while adding a pungent taste to boiling shellfish, pickling brines, marinades, game, venison, and stuffing.

MEDICINAL Laurel Bay tea is said to soothe the stomach, relieve the aches and pains associated with rheumatism, sprains, bruises, and skin rashes. There are indications that Bay Laurel leaves act as a mild sedative and a tea can be made before bedtime for better sleep.

MYSTICAL The burning of fresh Bay Laurel leaves is professed to increase psychic powers and for divination. A weak tea is said to increase wisdom and clairvoyance. If you are moving into a new home, or a vacant apartment, burning Bay Laurel leaves and letting the smoke linger in all four corners of the residence is said to purify the home and banish all evil. Place the leaves in a pillowcase for sleeping soundly and for prophetic dreams. If you write a wish on a Laurel Bay leaf, and then burn the leaf, your wish will come true.

BEE BALM (BERGAMOT, OSWEGO TEA, HORSEMINT)

Monarda didyma

Family	Lamiaceae – mint family
Origin	Eastern North America
Zones	A2, a3, 1-11, 14-17
Type	Herbaceous perennial
Inclination	Moderately invasive
Exposure	Full to half-sun; afternoon shade in hotter climates
Start	Cuttings, root divisions or seeds; seed sown flowers vary in color
Growth	To 3' x 1'
Flowers	Mid- to late-summer; colors include scarlet, red, pink, lavender, white and mixed shades of these colors; dried flowers are excellent for potpourri and in fresh and dry floral arrangements
Harvest	Leaves anytime but young leaves best
Fertilizer	Organic, all-purpose
Soil	Not particular
Tolerance	Will not tolerate cold, wet soils; deer resistant
Attracts	Bees, butterflies, and hummingbirds
Seaside	Yes; needs protection from wind
Containers	Yes

USES

CULINARY Leaves are used for tea and to season soups, salads, stews, etc. Literature suggests that pregnant women, and those with thyroid problems, should not ingest Bee Balm (Monarda).

MEDICINAL Oswego tea is a tasty, well-known remedy for digestive problems and appears to have beneficial properties in regard to improving appetite, relieving colic, reducing bloating, alleviating menstrual cramping, and reducing nausea and vomiting. The tea can also be used as a soothing drink to calm nerves. Bee Balm is often combined with other relaxants such as valerian and chamomile. Externally, the plants leaves can be used as an antiseptic and antibacterial ointment for use on minor wounds, insect stings, to help relieve eczema, psoriasis, cold sores and in the clearing up of acne. Deep breathing of steam from boiling leaves may help to relieve sore throat, fever, and congestion. Finally, Bee Balm can be used in aromatherapy. Put a handful of leaves in a mesh bag, or some hosiery, and run under hot bathwater for a relaxing, lemon scented bath.

MYSTICAL Carry a few leaves in your wallet to attract money, or rub leaves on the skin before an interview, or business meeting for success.

BORAGE

Borago officinalis

Family	Boraginaceae – Borage or Forget-Me-Not family
Origin	Europe
Zones	A2. A3, 1-24, h1
Type	Annual
Inclination	Non-invasive; may reseed under proper conditions
Exposure	Full to half-sun
Start	Seeds; place after all danger of frost has past; borage has a tap-root, so it does not transplant well
Growth	3' x 2'
Flowers	Blue, star shaped in hanging clusters summer through fall
Harvest	Flowers, stems, and leaves anytime; use fresh leaves as borage does not dry well; plant leaves impart a cucumber taste
Fertilizer	Organic
Soil	Rich, well-drained soil
Tolerance	Keep moist for best results; drought tolerant once established
Attracts	Bees
Seaside	Yes
Containers	Yes

USES

CULINARY — Borage flowers add a colorful garnish to salads, spreads, dips, and soups, and are also used as a garnish in drinks. The petals, leaves and stems add flavor to soups and stews when added during the last few minutes of cooking. The flowers can also be used as a floral cake decoration or can be candied.

MEDICINAL — Leaves are used in teas to help relieve depression, bronchitis and in reducing fevers. Borage also acts as an anti-diarrheal agent. Drink a cupful 2-3 times a day. Externally, grind the leaves into a paste to make a cooling, soothing remedy for sprains, swellings as well as skin irritations and inflammations. Borage leaves and flowers can be pulverized to make herbal capsules to take in lieu of tea.

MYSTICAL — Celtic warriors drank Borage flavored wine to give them courage in battle. Borage has also been recommended by herbalists throughout history as an effective anti-depressant, producing a feeling of elation. For courage, tuck a blossom in your pocket or purse before a stressful situation. Drinking Borage tea is also said to increase psychic powers.

CALENDULA (POT MARIGOLD)

Calendula officinalis

Family	Asteraceae – Aster family
Origin	Eastern Mediterranean
Zones	1-24, h1
Type	Annual
Inclination	Non-invasive; may reseed under proper conditions
Exposure	Full sun
Start	Seeds in spring, late summer, or early fall
Growth	2' x 2'
Flowers	Daisy-like bright orange and yellow flowers with shades of apricot, cream, and soft yellow, white or mixed. Dwarf strains are available; calendulas repel tomato hornworms and can be planted near tomatoes for this purpose; fragrant.
Harvest	Flowers and leaves
Fertilizer	Organic
Soil	Prefers well-drained soil; calendula grows best if planted with enriched soil as will produce better blossoms
Tolerance	Average water
Attracts	Bees
Seaside	Yes; subject to mildew in moist climates
Containers	Yes

USES

CULINARY — Flower petals can be used, fresh or dried, to add color to soups, stews, custards, omelets, cheeses and as a garnish. Petals are also used as a saffron substitute for rice. Leaves are bitter but can be used sparingly in soups and salads.

MEDICINAL — Make a powder for external use by drying the flowers, then grinding them and mixing with cornstarch or talc. An unsweetened tea rinse brings out highlights in blond and brunette hair. For a refreshing bath that helps the skin, tie a mesh bag, filled with flowers, under your bathtub faucet.

MYSTICAL — Ancient Egyptians valued Calendula for its alleged rejuvenation properties. The Greeks used it for a culinary garnish. The blossoms were woven into wreaths in India to decorate various images of their gods and goddesses. It has been reported that Civil War doctors used the leaves to treat open wounds on the battlefield. For protection, hang garlands over doors to prevent evil from entering your home. The petals can be scattered under the bed for prophetic dreams. Carry Calendula petals in your pocket or purse for a favorable outcome concerning legal matters. Taking a Calendula bath will garner you the respect and admiration of everyone you encounter. If a woman touches Calendula petals with her feet, she is supposed to be able to understand bird whistles and calls.

CARAWAY

Carum carvi

Family	Apiaceae – Carrot or Parsley family
Origin	Asia minor; usage dates back 5,000 years
Zones	1-24
Type	Biennial
Inclination	Non-invasive
Exposure	Full sun
Start	Seeds in early spring or fall; Caraway has a taproot and does not transplant well
Growth	2' x 1'
Flowers	White with a pink hue in umbrella like clusters that bloom after second year
Harvest	Flowers, leaves anytime (preferably young) and seeds in summer; dry flowers and seeds in a paper bag until seeds dry, then shake out and transfer to an airtight bag. Seeds are fragrant.
Container	Dried
Fertilizer	Organic
Soil	Well-drained and loose
Tolerance	Average water
Attracts	Bees – reputed to repel aphids, flies, and fruit moths in the garden, and helps to repel mosquitoes indoors
Seaside	Yes
Containers	Yes

USES

CULINARY Leaves can be used in soups and salads. Seeds are used on baked fruits, breads, cakes, cookies, dumplings, cream cheese, in stews, sauerkraut, soups, casseroles and goulashes. The root can be harvested, washed, and cooked like turnips or parsnips. For enhanced flavor, roast the Caraway seeds before using in cheese dishes or potato salad. Add Caraway in the last 15 minutes of cooking for best flavor.

MEDICINAL Make a tea to help alleviate gripe, stomach aches and digestive problems; up to four cups a day. Caraway seeds and oil improve gastric problems, flatulence, and indigestion. Use for relief of colic in young children. Crush an ounce of seed and let sit in cold water for about six hours. Sweeten if desired and administer 1-2 teaspoons up to four times a day. Also mash the seeds and place in a hot cloth to help with earaches. The mash can also be used to help heal bruises while the tea can be used as an expectorant.

MYSTICAL Carry the seeds in a sachet for protection from evil and to enhance memory. Place seeds under a child's bed to protect against disease. Carrying the seeds can also attract and help keep a lover. Caraway seeds made into a potion and fed to straying husbands will make them become faithful.

CATNIP

Nepeta cataria

Family	Lamiaceae – Mint family
Origin	Western Asia and Mediterranean
Zones	1-24
Type	Herbaceous perennial
Inclination	Reseeds under proper conditions
Exposure	Full to half-sun
Start	Cuttings before flower stalks form in spring, or seeds
Growth	To 3' x 2'
Flowers	Inconspicuous small, white to pink flowers in summer
Harvest	Harvest before flowers form; leaves anytime
Fertilizer	Organic, all-purpose
Soil	Light and well-drained
Tolerance	Average water
Attracts	Cats! And bees – bruising the leaves emits an odor that mimics a cats' sexual scent –therefore the attraction
Seaside	Yes
Containers	Yes

USES

CULINARY — Leaves can be used in salads and to flavor teas.

MEDICINAL — A tea can be used to help calm the nerves and help with insomnia. It is said to relieve colic in children and as a digestive aid for adults. Helps to alleviate gas, stomach cramps and nervousness in children, and is often considered the "children's herb." Catnip is often used in enemas to expel worms and restore the tone of bowels. Catnip has also been used for colds, dizziness, fevers, hysteria, morning sickness, small pox, and urine retention.

MYSTICAL — Catnip is reported to be related magically to animals, love, happiness, luck, and beauty. Growing Catnip will create a psychic bond between you and your cats. Use a sachet combined with rose petals to attract lovers. Inhale the steam from teas for beauty and happiness. Make some Catnip cookies, or candied Catnip, for all of the above.

CAYENNE PEPPER

Capsicum annum

Family	Solinaceae – Nightshade family
Origin	Tropical America
Zones	All zones
Type	Perennial in warm climates, annual in colder climates
Inclination	Non-invasive
Exposure	Full sun
Start	Seeds; plant indoors in early spring and set out after danger of frost has past; peppers need a long growing season (3-4 mos.) And temperatures consistently above 55° to set fruit
Growth	To 2' x 2'
Flowers	Inconspicuous, small white flowers
Harvest	When fruit turns red; the longer the peppers stay on the plant the hotter they will become
Fertilizer	Organic fruit and vegetable
Soil	Rich, well-drained soil for best results
Tolerance	Average water
Attracts	Salsa lovers!
Seaside	Not recommended
Containers	Yes

USES

CULINARY — While all peppers have culinary value, Cayenne also has special medicinal properties that set it apart from other peppers. Cayenne can be used to spice up oils and vinegars, as well as adding flavor to salsa, chili, dips, and the like. They can be added to pizza, barbeque sauces, scrambled eggs, stews, soups etc. for a spicy treat. Mature Cayenne peppers are packed with vitamins A and C, iron, potassium, calcium, and niacin.

MEDICINAL — Pregnant and lactating women should avoid Cayenne. Cayenne is professed to have soothing effects on the digestive system and to offer relief from colds, sore throats, fevers and to help increase circulation. A tea is also beneficial for hangovers. Dry peppers and grind them into a powder, using one or two tablespoons for relief, or put the powder into capsules for future use. Externally, Cayenne can be used to help relieve frostbite. A little on your hands and feet can help them keep warm. To make a liniment for external use, gently boil one tablespoon of powder with a pint of cider vinegar. Bottle the liquid while hot but do not strain. Make an oil and, using a cotton plug, saturate it in the oil and apply to a sore tooth cavity to help alleviate pain. Cayenne is also said to promote health to the heart and circulatory system.

MYSTICAL — Cayenne offers strength, courage, motivation, protection and increases one's aura. Do not burn Cayenne as incense as the vapors can induce violent sneezing.

CHAMOMILE, GERMAN

Matricaria recutita

Family	Asteraceae – Aster family
Origin	Western Asia and Europe
Zones	1-24
Type	Annual
Inclination	May reseed under proper conditions
Exposure	Full sun
Start	Seeds in early spring or fall; said to germinate better with recurrent freezing and thawing
Growth	To 2' x 1'
Flowers	Small, daisy-like, white and yellow to 1" wide; fragrant
Harvest	Flowers and young leaves; older leaves bitter and not usable
Fertilizer	Organic
Soil	Not particular but prefers well-drained soil
Tolerance	Keep soil moist, not wet
Attracts	Bees, birds, and butterflies
Seaside	Yes
Containers	Yes

USES

CULINARY Dried flowers are used for making the familiar, fragrant (similar to apples) Chamomile tea.

MEDICINAL Chamomile tea and capsules are used internally to help alleviate menstrual and stomach cramps, indigestion, flatulence, fever, colds, congestion, diarrhea, headaches, insomnia, vomiting, stress, depression, anxiety, nervousness, and poor digestion. For babies, it is helpful with colic and teething pain. The flowers can be used in bath water to ease hemorrhoid pain, and the oil can be applied to combat eczema and neuralgia. Chamomile flowers can be used in a steam inhaler for respiratory problems such as asthma, hay fever and sinusitis. For burns, dip a clean dressing in cooled tea and apply to wound. Most of all, Chamomile is used as a muscle relaxant. Two to three cups of tea a day, or two-three capsules a day, will usually suffice to help most ailments.

MYSTICAL Chamomile is tied to money, sleep, love, peace, purification, and tranquility. To attract a lover wash body, face and hair with bath water sweetened with Chamomile flowers. Also use Chamomile in your bath water for peace and tranquility when you are down and out. To increase your chances of winning at gambling, bathe your hands in Chamomile water. Place flowers in your pillow for a peaceful night's rest. Sprinkle the dried flowers around your property to protect from spells or curses. Chamomile is said to attract money by carrying the flowers with you or burning them in rituals.

CHERVIL (FRENCH PARSLEY)

Anthriscus cerefolium

Family	Apiaceae– Carrot or Parsley family
Origin	North Africa, Asia, and Europe
Zones	1-24
Type	Annual
Inclination	May reseed under proper conditions
Exposure	Part shade to three-quarters shade; does well indoors in well-lighted room
Start	Seeds in early spring or fall with mild winters, as plant goes to seed quickly in hotter climates; chervil has a taproot and does not transplant easily
Growth	To 2' x 2'
Flowers	Small, white umbrella like clusters; fragrant
Harvest	Flowers, leaves, and roots, which can be used fresh or dried; newer leaves give best results
Fertilizer	Organic
Soil	Well-drained
Tolerance	Keep soil moist, not wet
Attracts	Bees
Seaside	Yes
Containers	Yes

USES

CULINARY Chervil has an anise-parsley flavor and is closely related to parsley. Use it in vinegars, sauces, stews, soups, salads and with vegetables. Chervil can also be mixed with cheeses and butter and adds flavor to fish, chicken, and egg dishes. Dry Chervil quickly in an oven rather than the customary method of a dry, dark, and warm room. Chervil tends to go bitter with long cooking so it's best to add at the last minute.

MEDICINAL Chervil is best known as a remedy for high blood pressure. Make a tea or pulverize the dried leaves and use in capsules. The tea can also be used as an eye wash. Saturate a cotton ball and place it over the closed eye for approximately ten minutes. Chervil has also been used as a diuretic, expectorant, skin freshener, digestive aid and as a blood purifier. Chervil juice is good for the skin as a topical dressing. A strong Chervil tea, applied externally, will help alleviate the pain of insect bites as well as cuts and eczema. It can also be used in a facial mask for cleansing, deterring wrinkles and supporting skin resiliency. Fresh leaves in a warm poultice are supposed to ease aching joints. Chervil is a good source of vitamin C, carotene, iron, and magnesium.

MYSTICAL There is evidence of Chervil's use back to the ancient Egyptians. A basket of Chervil was found in Tutankhamen's tomb. Eating Chervil whole is said to cure hiccups.

CHICORY

Cichorium intybus

Family	Asteraceae – Aster family
Origin	Mediterranean; naturalized along U.S. west coast
Zones	All zones
Type	Herbaceous perennial
Inclination	Reseeds under proper conditions
Exposure	Full sun along coast; part shade inland; prefers cool weather
Start	Plant seeds spring or summer (where it's not too hot)
Growth	To 4' x 2'
Flowers	Sky blue flowers to 2" in diameter
Harvest	Leaves for salads; roots make a coffee substitute
Fertilizer	Organic
Soil	Well-drained
Tolerance	Drought tolerant once established
Attracts	Bees, butterflies, and flies
Seaside	Yes
Containers	Not recommended

USES

CULINARY Use leaves like lettuce in salads. Young roots can be boiled and eaten with butter. To make coffee, you will need to clean, roast, and grind the roots.

MEDICINAL As a tea Chicory is believed to treat jaundice and liver problems, as well as being helpful in relieving digestive disorders. Dip a cotton ball into some saved tea for a soothing eye wash. Mixed with honey it is useful as a mild laxative for children. Externally, bruise fresh leaves and apply to areas affected by skin lesions, swellings, gout, and rheumatism.

MYSTICAL Records of Chicory's usage date to ancient Egypt, Greece, and Rome. It is said to impart strength, divination, frugality, good luck and used to prevent frigidity as well as to open door locks, though you can only do this on St. James Day using a golden knife and some Chicory, the Chicory making you invisible on this day. Early settlers wore Chicory as a good luck charm, believing it removed obstacles on their journey's west.

CHERRY – WILD BLACK

Prunus serotina

Family	Rosacea – Rose family
Origin	Eastern United States; mountainous regions of Texas, New Mexico, and Arizona
Zones	4-8
Type	Deciduous tree
Inclination	Reseeds easily
Exposure	Full to ½ sun
Start	Cuttings or seeds
Growth	From 25' to 100' x 40'
Flowers	White, hanging clusters; fragrant
Harvest	Bark and fruit
Fertilizer	Organic, all-purpose
Soil	Well-drained
Tolerance	Drought tolerant once established
Attracts	Bees and birds
Seaside	Yes; requires protection from wind
Containers	No

USES

CULINARY — Fruit is bitter but can be used to make pies, jams, jellies, etc.

MEDICINAL — The inner bark has been used historically as a cough remedy, tonic and sedative.

MYSTICAL — None known.

CHICKWEED

Stellaria media

Family	Caryophyllaceae – Carnation family
Origin	Europe
Zones	Northern hemisphere
Type	Annual, biennial
Inclination	Invasive but easily controlled
Exposure	Full to half-sun
Start	Seeds – easy to propagate
Growth	To 8" x 1'
Flowers	White, star shaped
Harvest	Leaves and stems
Fertilizer	Organic
Soil	Not particular but does better in well-drained soil
Tolerance	Adapts to most conditions
Attracts	Bees and flies
Seaside	Yes
Containers	Yes

USES

CULINARY — Leaves are used in salads or you can cook the leaves and stems as a vegetable.

MEDICINAL — Internally, Chickweed is used for rheumatism, bronchitis, arthritis, menstrual pain, and pleurisy, in a decoction for constipation and as a blood builder. Externally, a Chickweed poultice is used for pluribus, joint inflammation, itchy skin, eczema, acne, hemorrhoids, varicose veins, psoriasis, inflammations, ulcers, vaginitis, urticaria, boils, abscesses, allergies, and other skin problems.

MYSTICAL — Chickweed teaches us how to live and survive in balance with ourselves and others.

CHIVES

Allium schoenoprasum

Family	Amaryllidaceae – Amaryllis family
Origin	Europe
Zones	All zones
Type	Herbaceous perennial
Inclination	Non-invasive
Exposure	Full to ½ sun
Start	Divisions in spring or seeds
Growth	To 2' x 1'
Flowers	Rose-purple blooms in spring and summer; use in dried flower arrangements
Harvest	Flowers and stems anytime; snap off stems at base, rather than cut, as cuts will leave brown marks; flowers are also edible when first forming
Fertilizer	Organic
Soil	Not particular but prefers well-drained, organically enriched soil
Tolerance	Drought tolerant once established; however, does better with regular watering; deer resistant
Attracts	Bees
Seaside	Yes
Containers	Yes

USES

CULINARY — Use Chives in herbal vinegars, cheeses, butters to flavor salads, potatoes, soups, fish, scrambled eggs, and meats. Flowers can be used as a garnish or in your salad.

MEDICINAL — A paste or ointment made from Chives is said to prevent infection in burns and wounds. Mix the juice from squeezed stems with vinegar externally to reduce age spots, freckles, and warts. Chives are a member of the onion family and eating same is said to have some impact on high cholesterol and high blood pressure. Including them in your diet on a regular basis is said to help control those problems.

MYSTICAL — Sprinkling Chives juice on your head, when sitting in the sun, is said to cure baldness. Oh, yeah!

CILANTRO (CORIANDER)

Coriandrum sativum

Family	Apiacea – Carrot or Parsley family
Origin	Mediterranean
Zones	All zones
Type	Annual
Inclination	Non-invasive; cilantro is more difficult than most herbs to grow as it is short lived and needs cool temperatures to do well; keep roots as cool as possible with heavy mulching
Exposure	Full sun in cooler climates; light shade in warm climates
Start	Seeds in spring; sow in place as plants are difficult to transplant
Growth	To 2' x 1'
Flowers	Flat clusters of pinkish-white flowers bloom in summer
Harvest	Flowers, leaves, and seeds; begin harvesting leaves about one month after plant germinates; harvest seeds when mature
Soil	Rich and well-drained
Tolerance	Average water
Attracts	Bees and butterflies
Seaside	Yes; needs protection from wind
Containers	Yes

USES

CULINARY — Cilantro, like basil, is one of the more widely used herbs worldwide. The leaves and seeds are used to enhance soups, stews, salads, salsas, etc.

MEDICINAL — For an upset stomach and flatulence relief chew seeds or drink a tea made from the seeds. To help relieve the pain of rheumatism pound the seeds, add hot water to make a paste, and then apply to the affected area. For a thicker consistency oatmeal can be added.

MYSTICAL — Cilantro has been used since ancient times as an aphrodisiac. Carry a sachet on your person, or use powdered seeds in warm wine, or beer, to attract the one you love. Hanging stems and flowers in all corners of the house is said to offer protection and keep away unwanted guests. Burn as incense for the same effect. Cilantro has been associated with immortality for centuries. Drinking Cilantro tea is said to help ease the pain of a relationship break-up. Put some seeds or leaves in your pillowcase for a safe, protected sleep.

CONEFLOWER (ECHINACEAE)

Echinaceae purpurea

Family	Asteraceae – Aster family
Origin	Central and eastern North America
Zones	A2, a3, 1-24
Type	Herbaceous perennial
Inclination	Non-invasive; may reseed under proper conditions
Exposure	Full to half-sun
Start	Divisions in fall and winter or seeds in spring
Growth	To 2' x 2'; flower stalks to 3'- 4'
Flowers	Pink, rose, purple, white, dark red with orange to yellow cones summer and fall
Harvest	Rhizomes and roots anytime
Fertilizer	Organic, all-purpose
Soil	Well-drained
Tolerance	Some drought tolerance once established
Attracts	Bees and butterflies; seeds are a favorite of finches
Seaside	Yes
Containers	Yes

USES

CULINARY — None known.

MEDICINAL — Coneflower has long been known as one of nature's most beneficial medicinal plants. As an ointment Coneflower can be used for treatment of insect bites, burns, measles, skin ulcers, herpes, sores, cold sores, yeast infections in women and infected injuries. It is purportedly effective against anti-venom snakebites. As a tea it is said to reduce symptoms of a scratchy or sore throat, stomach cramps, urinary tract infections, lymph node inflammation and cold or flu symptoms. Coneflower is perhaps best known for its properties that boost the human immune system and for skin healing, fungal infections, and psoriasis. It is also used to help in fighting rabies, venereal diseases, ear infections and septicemia.

MYSTICAL — According to legend, Native Americans used the rhizome, when chewed on, to induce numbing sensations in the feet, hands, and throat, lessening pain and allowing them to walk on hot coals, as well as handling and swallowing hot items.

DANDELION

Taraxacum officinale

Family	Asteraceae – Aster family
Origin	Asia, Europe, and North America; naturalized worldwide
Zones	All zones
Type	Perennial
Inclination	Invasive; sows readily
Exposure	Full to half-sun
Start	Seeds in spring, summer or fall
Growth	To 2" x 1' - flower stalks to 1'
Flowers	Yellow
Harvest	Leaves when young or in fall; tap roots harvested fall through spring
Fertilizer	Any
Soil	Prefers well-drained, moist soil
Tolerance	Drought tolerant once established
Attracts	Bees and butterflies
Seaside	Yes
Containers	Yes

USES

CULINARY Dandelion plants are perhaps one of the most maligned plants on our planet, yet, if utilized, one of the best herbs for human use. They are high in vitamins A and C with healthy doses of beta carotene, potassium, iron, copper, and other vitamins. Use fresh leaves (cut before flowers bud) in salads or cook like spinach — harvest tap root without breaking and roast in an oven set at 250°. Turn occasionally until dry but not burned — once roasted cut into chunks and add to soups, stews, pastas, casseroles, vegetable dishes or grind and use for Dandelion coffee. Ground roots mixed with warm milk and a little sweetener makes a tasty and nutritious beverage with few calories. Dandelion wine is made from the flowers and Dandelion tea from the leaves.

MEDICINAL Dandelions are considered safe and effective as a general tonic that helps strengthen the gallbladder, pancreas, spleen, liver, stomach, and intestines while helping to reduce inflammation in hepatitis and cirrhosis. They are also believed to help dissipate gallstones and improve kidney function. As a tea it is helpful in relieving constipation, digestive disorders, indigestion, sluggishness, and fatigue. The tea may also be beneficial for problems associated with diabetes and low blood sugar. Externally, the white sap from roots and stems can be applied directly to ease the pain of sores and insect bites and is said to help eliminate warts, acne, and calluses.

MYSTICAL If you blow hard on a seed head, and all the seeds blow off, your wish will come true. If a woman eliminates all the seed heads, then her lover loves only her. If seeds stay on, he is not loyal. Blow (not too hard!) on a seed head and the number of seeds left will tell you how many children you are going to have. If you see seeds falling off the flower head, when there is no wind, rain is on the way. Also, when you blow on a seed head the number of seeds left will tell you how many years you have left to live. The list goes on and on. The roots and leaves can be made into teas for spells and rituals concerning divination, calling spirits, psychic powers and wishes. Parts of the plant thrown together in a sachet, or worn around the neck in a small, flannel bag, are supposed to help wishes come true.

DILL

Anethum graveolens

Family	Apiaceae – Carrot or Parsley family
Origin	Southwestern Asia and southern Europe; naturalized in northern United States
Zones	1-24
Type	Annual
Inclination	Seeds sow readily under proper conditions
Exposure	Full to half-sun
Start	Seeds in spring; in hotter climates, sow seeds in mid-summer for fall and winter harvest
Growth	To 4' x 2'
Flowers	Small, yellow, umbrella like wide clusters to 6" wide
Harvest	Leaves and seeds; leaves any time before plant bears flowers. Leaves can be dried but keep their flavor better by first freezing and then thawing; seeds can be harvested three weeks after flowers blossom
Fertilizer	Organic
Soil	Moderately rich, well-drained
Tolerance	Keep moist, not wet for best results; deer resistant
Attracts	Bees
Seaside	Yes; needs protection from wind
Containers	Yes

USES

CULINARY Leaves and seeds are used to flavor vinegars and mustard-based sauces and dressings. Dill is also used to flavor fish, tomatoes, lamb, shellfish, eggs, pickles, sandwiches, and salads as well as other meats and vegetables.

MEDICINAL Dill can be used to soothe the stomach and as an anti-gas remedy. It is also said to increase mother's milk and help treat breast congestion. Use for colic in children, indigestion or for help in healing skin sores and rashes.

MYSTICAL Dill is used in love and lust charms as well as sachets. Placing the seeds in a muslin bag under your shower, or in your bath water, is said to protect your home, and you, from harm. There is a history of dill being used as far back as biblical times.

EVENING PRIMROSE

Oenothera hookeri

Family	Onagraceae – Evening Primrose family
Origin	Asia, Europe, and western United States; naturalizes in moist climates
Zones	5-7, 14-24
Type	Perennial
Inclination	Invasive
Exposure	Full to half-sun
Start	Root divisions in spring or seeds in fall and spring
Growth	To 3'- 6' x 2'
Flowers	Yellow flowers turn to orange-red on tall, hairy stems; flowers bloom all summer into fall, and are very prolific; flowers open in the evening and close in the morning; fragrant
Harvest	Flowers, leaves, and roots anytime
Fertilizer	Not particular
Soil	Prefers rich, moist, and well-drained soil
Tolerance	Both drought and flood resistant
Attracts	Bees, birds, and butterflies
Seaside	Yes
Containers	Not recommended

USES

CULINARY Leaves, roots, and flowers can be added to salads.

MEDICINAL Reduces or eliminates many problems associated with PMS, including irritability, depression, bloating, and breast pain. If taken regularly, Evening Primrose is purported to regulate menstrual periods and, in fact, in Europe, the oil is already established as an excellent remedy for PMS. Taken as a tea it helps fight obesity. Other problems for which the oil (taken internally) is used include asthma, cholesterol regulation, arteriosclerosis, prostate health, allergies, headaches, and rheumatoid arthritis, multiple sclerosis, lupus, and scleroderma. Also, the oil helps alleviate complications arising from diabetes including numbness, tingling and poor circulation as well as treating cirrhosis of the liver. Externally the leaves, stems, and roots, used as a tea, are nourishing for the skin, and is used in treatment of acne, dry skin, rashes, itchiness, eczema and for overall skin health. Eating the flowers, leaves, or roots, provides the same health benefits as taking commercial oil preparations. Native Americans used Evening Primrose to treat stomach aches, hemorrhoids, sore throats, and scrapes.

MYSTICAL None known.

FENNEL

Foeniculum vulgare

Family	Apiaceae – Carrot or Parsley family
Origin	South Africa, China, central and western Europe
Zones	All zones
Type	Herbaceous perennial; treated as a summer annual in colder zones and winter annual in hotter climates
Inclination	Non-invasive, except in mildest climates; may self-sow elsewhere under proper conditions
Exposure	Full to half-sun
Start	Seeds in spring; as fennel does not transplant well, plant seeds in desired locations
Growth	To 3'–5' x 2'; Florence fennel to 2' x 1'
Flowers	Yellow umbrella like flat clusters in summer; fragrant
Harvest	Leaves and stems anytime; seeds after turning brown
Fertilizer	Not particular
Soil	Light and well-drained
Tolerance	Drought tolerant once established, but performs better with regular watering
Attracts	Bees, birds, and butterflies – fennel is a host for the swallowtail butterfly
Seaside	Yes; requires protection from wind
Containers	Not recommended except for Florence variety

USES

CULINARY Fennel is popular in French and Italian cuisine. Its leaves can be used with fish, veal, and pork as well as mixed with butters, cheeses, oils, sauces, vinegars, and salad dressings. The seeds can be used as a spice for breads, cakes, cookies, and other baked products and added to cabbage, beets, pickles, lentils, and potatoes for added flavor. Fennel is also used as a fragrance for soaps and perfumes.

MEDICINAL Fennel is an appetite depressant and was used during Medieval times (on church fasting days) to deter hunger and was also used as a breath freshener. A tea is recommended to increase the flow of milk in nursing mothers and ease symptoms associated with menopause. Leaves and stems can be pounded into a paste and used to relieve breast swelling. Fennel teas have been used throughout history to quiet hiccups, prevent nausea, break up kidney stones, aid digestion, prevent gout, purify the liver, reverse alcohol damage to the liver, and to treat jaundice. Fennel is also used as a flea repellent around the house and in pet bedding as well as a cleansing herb. It has also been used as a steam facial for opening pores and rejuvenating facial skin.

MYSTICAL Fennel is said to have been discovered by the Greeks and spread around the Old World by the Romans. To attain longevity, fertility, healing, love, clairvoyance, purification, and strength drink Fennel as a tea or carry a sachet on your person. This will also prevent negativity and provide protection from harmful spells. When casting a spell Fennel can be used to impart courage, divination, cleansing, energy, meditation, virility, psychic protection and used to counter someone else's magic. Hang in doorways or windows to protect your home from evil and sorcery. Placed in keyholes it is said to protect your home from dead spirits. Grown around the home Fennel provides protection from negativity and evil influences.

FEVERFEW

Chrysanthemum parthenium

Family	Chrysanthemum – Daisy family
Origin	Eurasia – has naturalized in North America
Zones	1-24, a1
Type	Herbaceous perennial
Inclination	Non-invasive; however, may self-sow easily under proper conditions
Exposure	Full to half-sun
Start	Clumps, cuttings, or divisions anytime; seeds in early spring
Growth	To 2' x 1'
Flowers	Small, white flowers in dense clusters
Harvest	Flowers and leaves anytime
Fertilizer	Not particular
Soil	Prefers well-drained soil
Tolerance	Somewhat drought resistance once established
Attracts	Nothing – repels bees and other insects – good insect repellant around tomatoes, etc.; deer resistant
Seaside	Yes
Containers	Yes

USES

CULINARY None known.

MEDICINAL If you don't want bees on your porch, or around your outdoor dining tables, you can plant Feverfew in containers to help drive them away. Similarly, if you want bees in your garden or for your crops, you need Feverfew to keep its distance. Despite its name, there is little basis to support the claim that it is effective in helping to reduce fevers. However, it has been scientifically proven to help relieve migraines, arthritis pain, rheumatism, and muscle spasms. It is also purported to be used as an anti-gas agent, a digestive aid and to help control painful menstruation. Feverfew leaves and flowers have a bitter taste, so don't eat more that 3-4 leaves a day, or add them to your salad to help diminish the taste. Leaves and flowers can be dried and used in capsules, or you can freeze the leaves for later use. Externally, fresh leaves can be rubbed on the skin, or made into an ointment for protection from biting and stinging insects. The leaves can also be used in this manner to help relieve itching skin.

MYSTICAL Worn around the neck, or carried in your purse, pocket or suitcase, Feverfew is purported to protect from accidents, injury, and sickness. When ingested as a tea, Feverfew protects from flu, cold and fevers. Feverfew is used to promote spiritual healing, for use in meditation, to help you relax and to promote love or cast a spell. Use Feverfew in sachets and charms.

GARLIC

Allium sativum

Family	Amaryllidacaea – Onion family
Origin	Southern Europe; different, less desirable varieties grow worldwide
Zones	All zones, except a1
Type	Perennial
Inclination	Non-invasive
Exposure	Full sun recommended but tolerates some shade
Start	Seeds (slow) or cloves in spring; best to buy cloves from reputable nurseries or seed companies as store-bought varieties may have been sprayed with harmful pesticides or preservatives; can plant in fall in mild winter areas for harvest the following fall
Growth	To 1' x 1'; flower stalks to 2'
Flowers	Attractive, light to dark blue flowers on stalks; used in dried flower arrangements
Harvest	In fall, when leafy tops fall over,; lift out bulbs with a garden fork, rather than pulling them out. Air dry the bulbs after cutting off most of the tops and roots, then store in a cool, dry place on a screen or braid (leaving leaves and stalks on) and hang in a cool, dry place
Fertilizer	Organic
Soil	Well-drained
Tolerance	Drought resistant but better with regular water; be careful not to overwater; deer resistant
Attracts	Bees
Seaside	Yes
Containers	Yes

USES

CULINARY   Garlic can be, and is, used (according to taste) in about every dish (i.e., soups, salads, stews, with meat and vegetables) known to man, except desserts.

MEDICINAL   Garlic is one of the safest herbs to use medicinally but has its well-known odor as a drawback. Garlic contains a substance called *Allicin*, which has properties similar to weak penicillin. Garlic is used as a remedy for many ailments, which has a long list, including wounds, ulcers, some viruses, skin infections, flu, strep throat, worms, high blood pressure and respiratory ailments. It is purported to help with stomach cancer as well as colic, colds, kidney, and bladder problems along with ear aches to name a few. Garlic is also believed to cure worms in dogs if you can get them to swallow it.

MYSTICAL   Garlic has been believed to possess magical properties for centuries. If you carry cloves with you while on the water, you will not drown. Peeled cloves placed in doorways and around the house is said to keep evil and illness at bay, particularly in new homes. A clove under the pillows of children will protect them while sleeping. By placing a garlic bulb, with two crossed pins stuck in it, at a road intersection, you can ditch a former lover. If you can lure him, or her, to stand over the clove, they will lose interest in you. Eating, or carrying Garlic on your person, is said to enhance speed, strength, endurance and courage, and soldiers throughout history have used it when going into battle. By the same token, Garlic was given to slaves to protect them from disease and enhance strength. Rub a cut clove over a sore or other skin ailment, then place the disturbance under running water to wash away the ailment.

GINKGO (MAIDENHAIR TREE)

Ginkgo biloba

Family	Ginkgoaceae – related to conifers – ginkgo family
Origin	China; 200 million years ago -this plant purportedly grew around the world
Zones	A3, 1-10, 12, 14-24
Type	Deciduous tree
Inclination	Non-invasive; female trees messy – planting only male trees recommended
Exposure	Full to half-sun for best fall color; tolerates shady places
Start	Softwood cuttings in mid-summer
Growth	To 70' x 35'; slow to moderate growth
Flowers	Inconspicuous, yellow flowers on females, and greenish-yellow catkins on males, which bloom April-May
Harvest	Pick leaves when fresh and let dry before using
Fertilizer	Not particular
Soil	Deep and loose, well-drained soil
Tolerance	Some drought tolerance once established; deer resistant
Attracts	Bees
Seaside	Yes
Containers	Yes; makes an excellent bonsai tree

USES

CULINARY — None known.

MEDICINAL — Ginkgo has been proven to increase blood circulation to the entire body and, as such, sometimes labeled an anti-aging agent. Dry fresh Ginkgo leaves and use in tea or make into capsules. The plants leaves are used by older people as an energizer to improve mood, memory, attention span and alertness. Ginkgo appears to protect veins and arteries, preserving their tone and elasticity. Ginkgo is used as a remedy for many ailments including dementia, Alzheimer's, arteriosclerosis, peripheral vascular diseases, peripheral neuropathy, and overall poor blood circulation. The plant appears to have had some success in helping with macular degeneration and, subsequently, help with tinnitus and vertigo. Less documented improvements are relief from hangovers, impotence in males and increased sex drive in both males and females, i.e., something of an aphrodisiac. Gingko has powerful antioxidant properties making it a possible good choice for prevention, and possible reversal, of stroke damage, cardiovascular problems, and occlusive arterial disease. It has also been used to ease inflammations caused by asthma and allergies and relieves symptoms associated with multiple sclerosis. Best of all, minimal side effects are associated with the usage of Ginkgo, and this plant has been said to be mankind's closest thing to the Fountain of Youth.

MYSTICAL — Because the venation in Ginkgo leaves somewhat resemble the human brain, this herb has been used as a "brain food" for centuries. Because it thrived during the age of dinosaurs and has maintained its basic properties down through the ages, the Maidenhair Tree is considered magical by many races of man. Ginkgo is considered to have high magical energy and is used in longevity and age spells. A tradition long held, for a healthy and prosperous life, is to plant a Ginkgo tree when someone you know has been born, and upon their death to insure their place in the afterlife.

GINSENG, AMERICAN

Panax quinquefolius

Family	Araliaceae – Aralia family
Origin	America and Korea; for Asian and Chinese ginseng look for *Panax ginseng*
Zones	Most woodlands and forests with cold winters
Type	Herbaceous perennial
Inclination	Non-invasive; self-pollinating
Exposure	Shade to deep shade
Start	Seeds in fall
Growth	To 3' x 4' x 1'
Flowers	Small, greenish-white (not showy) flowers with attractive red berries in fall
Harvest	Roots in fall; takes about 6-7 years in soil for plants to grow big enough to harvest; use a garden fork and remove gently from soil, then clean and place on a screen in shade to dry, or dry indoors; turn regularly and watch for mold; roots are ready to use when thoroughly dry; seeds can still be planted after 3-4 years
Fertilizer	Organic
Soil	Requires excellent drainage as is susceptible to many rots and funguses
Tolerance	Keep moist but not wet
Attracts	Deer
Seaside	Not recommended
Containers	Yes

USES

CULINARY Ingested as a tea, Ginseng is believed to be a powerful aphrodisiac. To prepare tea, boil two cups of water in a non-metallic container and remove from heat. Steep a slice of Ginseng root (or three teaspoons powder, or one tea bag) and cover at least five minutes. Flavor to taste with sugar, honey, or whatever suits you.

MEDICINAL Ginseng is purported to be an energizer and stress reducer and appears to benefit both high and low blood pressure. It improves mental clarity and memory, enhances physical stamina, and bolsters the immune system. Studies have shown it can normalize blood sugar in Type 2 diabetes and helps cure insomnia and chest congestion associated with wheezing, persistent coughing, and shortness of breath. It is said to strengthen the heart, lungs, spleen, liver, kidneys, and pancreas and is therefore considered to be something of an anti-aging herb by improving overall health. One of the best recommended ways to use Ginseng is to just eat it uncooked, but you can make tea or capsules from it.

MYSTICAL The alleged magical powers of Ginseng date back thousands of years. Legend has it that these plants mysteriously rise from the ground at night and, glowing, flit about the forest floor, perhaps giving rise to fairy tales and the like. The forked root of the plant gives the impression of a human figure, giving rise to the aphrodisiac qualities associate with it. Ginseng "legs," with an appendage between the two legs, are considered the most valuable roots of all. In that regard, Ginseng is highly prized as a tonic that promotes sexual potency, vitality, lust, and long life. Ginseng root is carried on one's person to attract love, money and to enhance beauty. Ginseng also provides protection, grants wishes and enhances spirituality. Burning Ginseng root or powder is believed to ward off evil, break hexes or curses and repel negative spirits.

GOLDENROD

Solidago canadensis

Family	Asteraceae – Aster family
Origin	Eastern United States
Zones	1-11, 14-23
Type	Herbaceous perennial
Inclination	Invasive; may self-sow under proper conditions
Exposure	Full to half-sun
Start	Root division or seeds
Growth	To 3'- 4' x 2'
Flowers	Large, branching clusters of small, bright yellow flowers; excellent cut flowers with longevity
Harvest	Young leaves and root divisions anytime; seeds in fall
Fertilizer	Generally, not necessary; use fertilizer sparingly (if at all)
Soil	Not particular; does better with some cultivation
Tolerance	Average water; drought tolerant once established; deer resistant
Attracts	Bees, birds, and butterflies
Seaside	Yes
Containers	Yes

USES

CULINARY Leaves smell like anise when crushed and make a welcome anise-flavored tea. Goldenrod dried leaves can also be used as a top dressing for cakes, cookies, etc.

MEDICINAL Contrary to popular opinion, Goldenrod does not cause hay fever or allergies. In fact, it has been used to treat the two aliments. Internally, Goldenrod has been practical in treating kidney stones, urinary tract infections, digestive problems, bladder inflammation, colds, and the flu along with sore throats, laryngitis, and fatigue. Externally, Native Americans boiled the leaves and used them as an astringent and an antiseptic for wounds, eczema, arthritis, and rheumatism. Goldenrod is widely accepted in European countries as a remedy for bladder problems and kidney stones, and as a diuretic to help flush out urinary tract infections. Blue Mountain Tea, as it is called by herbalists in the Appalachian Mountains, has been used by residents of the region to relieve exhaustion and fatigue for years.

MYSTICAL Goldenrod is right up there as a love potion. Carry the flowers of Goldenrod around with you for a day and your future boyfriend or girlfriend will show up the day after. Goldenrod tea given to your lover is supposed to increase their love for you. Burn or crush leaves, or flowers, to help you in your pursuit of love. A stalk of Goldenrod is often used as a dowsing rod to search for lost objects or treasure. The flowers will nod in the direction of what you are seeking. Drinking Goldenrod tea keeps you in tune with yourself and helps you focus on your future. Planted near your doorstep, Goldenrod is said to increase your chance for peace, love, and prosperity in the future. If a plant sprouts near your front door, on its own, your luck will increase.

GOLDENSEAL

Hydrastis canadensis

Family	Ranuculaceae – Buttercup family
Origin	Northeastern United States
Zones	3-7
Type	Herbaceous perennial
Inclination	Non-invasive
Exposure	Full to partial shade
Start	Divisions or seeds
Growth	To 18" x 18"
Flowers	Greenish-white
Harvest	Seeds
Fertilizer	Compost and organics
Soil	Rich in organic material
Tolerance	Average water; deer resistant
Attracts	Bees and butterflies
Seaside	Yes
Containers	Yes

USES

CULINARY — None known.

MEDICINAL — Goldenseal is used as a topical antimicrobial herb, and as a means to remove canker sores when gargled. Herbalists also consider Goldenseal to be anti-inflammatory, antiseptic, astringent, anti-diabetic and used as both a laxative and as a muscular stimulant. Goldenseal is very bitter, which increases appetite, aids digestion, and often stimulates bile secretion. It has been used successfully to fight e-coli bacteria. The Cherokee mixed a powder from the root with bear fat for use as an insect repellent. It was used as a cancer treatment, an ophthalmic wash, as a yellow dye and as a remedy for stomachaches, wounds, whooping cough, and pneumonia.

MYSTICAL — Contrary to hearsay and some old-time legends, Goldenseal does not mask any traces of marijuana in your bloodstream.

HOREHOUND

Marrubium vulgare

Family	Lamiaceae – Mint family
Origin	Western Asia and Mediterranean region; naturalized in many parts of the world
Zones	1-24
Type	Herbaceous perennial
Inclination	Invasive
Exposure	Full to half-sun
Start	Cuttings spring to summer; root divisions or seeds in spring
Growth	To 3' x 2'
Flowers	Rounded whorls of white (not showy); leaves make attractive decorations in living and dry floral arrangements
Harvest	Leaves only, anytime
Fertilizer	Organic preferred
Soil	Not particular – the better the soil, the better the plant
Tolerance	Drought resistant once established; deer resistant
Attracts	Bees
Seaside	Yes
Containers	Yes

USES

CULINARY — Leaves are used to make tea, candy, and cough syrup.

MEDICINAL — Horehound is an effective immune booster and is quite nutritious containing vitamins A, B, C and E, essential fatty acids, iron, potassium and marrubin, an expectorant. Indeed, Horehound has been considered the champion of herbs for chest problems for thousands of years. Horehound is effective in loosening phlegm and mucus in the bronchial tubes and in the lungs. It also helps in relieving sore throats, coughs, and laryngitis.

MYSTICAL — Ancient herbalists prescribed Horehound for fevers, malaria and as an antidote for snakebites. It is traditionally carried in sachets for protection against sorcery and, when mixed with ash leaves and placed in a bowl of water by a sick person, Horehound is said to release healing vibrations. As a tea, the herb is supposed to promote mental acumen and clarity.

HYSSOP

Hyssopus officinalis

Family	Lamiaceae – Mint family
Origin	Southern Europe; Romans are believed to have introduced plant to Britain
Zones	1-24
Type	Herbaceous perennial
Inclination	Non-invasive; however, may self-sow under proper conditions
Exposure	Full to half-sun
Start	Cuttings or divisions in summer and fall; sow seeds in early spring, ¼ inch deep
Growth	To 2' x 3'
Flowers	Profusion of dark blue spikes in summer and fall; white, pink, and lavender varieties also available; fragrant
Harvest	Flowers can be used but do not use woody parts of plants; peppery tasting leaves sometimes used in cooking; harvest when leaves are tender
Fertilizer	Organic
Soil	Light, dry, rocky, well-drained
Tolerance	Some drought tolerance once established; deer resistant
Attracts	Bees, butterflies, and hummingbirds
Seaside	Yes
Containers	Yes

USES

CULINARY — Tender leaves can be used sparingly in salads, marinades, and stews while both leaves and seeds can be used with poultry stuffing, in chicken soup, apple pies, on cookies, etc. and the leaves can be dried for teas.

MEDICINAL — Internally, Hyssop can be used as a tea to remedy bronchitis, as an expectorant, and as a gargle for sore throats. Externally, the leaves can be made into an ointment. This can be used for treating muscular rheumatism, cuts, scrapes, bruises, cold sores, herpes sores, to heal scars, and is said to help strengthen the immune system. To make a Hyssop compress use one ounce of herb to one pint of boiling water. Let steep for 30 minutes, cover and let cool. Next, soak a clean cloth in the liquid and apply. Ideal for stomach aches, hemorrhoids, sore throats, and scrapes.

MYSTICAL — Hyssop is what is known as a purifying herb. It has a camphor-like odor and has long been known as a cleansing herb. As far back as the Seventh Century, Hyssop is purported to have been used as an air freshener in sickrooms and kitchens. When placed in the house, around windows and doors, it is supposed to protect your home from harm. Sprinkle Hyssop oil around your home to protect it or use in purification and healing baths by putting the leaves in a bag under running water. Hyssop has long been associated with dragons. Burn as an incense, or throw the leaves into a fire, to gain the power of dragons.

LAVENDER, ENGLISH

Lavandula angustifolia (officinalis)

Family	Lamiaceae – Mint family
Origin	Mediterranean region; usage began around 2500-4000 years ago
Zones	2-24
Type	Evergreen perennial; hardiest and most widely planted of species
Inclination	Non-invasive; however, may self-sow under proper conditions
Exposure	Full to half-sun
Start	Cuttings in spring and summer or seeds in spring ; there are many species of lavender with differences in height, width and flower color, so select the species you want from Sunset Magazine, other gardening books or online sites; with all the cross breeding, should you decide to propagate a plant you like from seed, chances are good you won't get the plant you wanted
Growth	Generally, 2'-3' x 2' but varies from species to species
Flowers	Generally, Lavender is purple, however white, pink and yellow varieties are available
Harvest	Flowers in late summer
Fertilizer	Not required (but a little won't hurt)
Soil	Well-drained
Tolerance	Drought tolerant once established; deer resistant
Attracts	Bees and butterflies
Seaside	Yes
Containers	Yes

USES

CULINARY — Make a téa from Lavender flowers to promote relaxation, peace, health, longevity, protection, and love. As an edible herb, Lavender can be blended with other herbs in meat and cheese dishes. Lavender can also be used to flavor vinegars, jellies, and ice cream. Like Hyssop and Anise, English Lavender yields a quality honey for beekeepers, and the flowers can also be candied and used for cake decorations.

MEDICINAL — Lavender is perhaps the all-time leader in herbs for medicinal properties. Records of its usage date back several centuries. Taken internally as a tea (or mixed with cookie dough, etc.), it has been beneficial for reducing stress, anxiety, exhaustion, irritability, headaches, migraines, insomnia, depression, colds, digestion, flatulence, upset stomach, liver and gall bladder problems, nervousness, and loss of appetite. Externally, use the unsweetened tea as a hair rinse to help reduce hair loss and dandruff. Dried stems, stripped of their leaves, can be burned as incense, or use them for basket weaving and making Lavender wands. Lavender oil is also used as an antiseptic and for aromatherapy.

Today the oil is also used as a base ingredient in many perfumes, soaps, shaving creams, cleaning supplies and scents. The dried flowers are added to dresser drawers and bathroom cupboards, and elsewhere, to freshen clothing and repel moths. Many cosmetics, such as lotions, lip balms and bath salts, contain Lavender's essential oils too.

MYSTICAL — According to history, the dried flowers were, and still are, often included in rituals, and spells, to attract a lover, and used to attract money as well. The flowers are also used in sleep and dream pillows, potpourris, and sachets to help you get a good night's rest, and for good health and luck.

LEMON BALM

Melissa officinalis

Family	Lamiaceae – Mint family
Origin	Southern Europe
Zones	1-24
Type	Herbaceous perennial
Inclination	Invasive
Exposure	Full to half-sun
Start	Cuttings in spring and summer, divisions anytime, or seeds in spring and summer
Growth	To 2' x 6'; aggressive groundcover
Flowers	Inconspicuous white to lavender-white flowers on spikes
Harvest	Flowers anytime; leaves before plants start to flower but best with new growth
Fertilizer	Not particular
Soil	Rich and moist preferred but will tolerate many conditions
Tolerance	Will tolerate both drought and wet conditions
Attracts	Bees and butterflies
Seaside	Yes
Containers	Best due to invasive nature

USES

CULINARY — Leaves can be used fresh, dried, or ground and are useful for cold and hot drinks, fruit cups, green salads, poultry, and stuffing along with fish marinades and dishes. Dried leaves are useful in sachets and potpourris or use Lemon Balm to help flavor wines or as a garnish in soups. Make a tasteful tea from its leaves or add leaves to other teas for a refreshing drink.

MEDICINAL — Lemon Balm has been used for centuries as a mild form of drug similar to Valium. It is also considered valuable as a virus and bacteria inhibitor so try using it for cleaning sores, scrapes, and cuts. It is also purported to induce sweating to help break fevers and for regulating menses.

MYSTICAL — It is said that if you carry Lemon Balm in a charm or sachet, it will help you find love. If you drink a tea made from the plant, it will help ease the pain after a bad relationship. Lemon Balm has been used for spells associated with healing, health, friendship, love, and success.

LEMON GRASS

Cymbopogon citratus

Family	Poaceae – Grass family
Origin	India and Malaysia
Zones	12, 13, 16, 17, 23, 24 h1, h2; bring indoors in winter in other zones and protect from cold weather below 45°
Type	Perennial
Inclination	Non-invasive
Exposure	Full to half-sun
Start	Divisions anytime; seeds anytime in above zones, spring elsewhere
Growth	To 3' - 4' x 2' in mild climates; to 6' x 3' or higher in tropical locations
Flowers	Inconspicuous, white
Harvest	Leaves and stalks anytime
Fertilizer	Compost or high nitrogen fertilizer; best with combination
Soil	Average to highly organic
Tolerance	Always keep moist; grows in bog conditions
Attracts	Unknown, but repels insects, including mosquitoes
Seaside	Yes
Containers	Yes

USES

CULINARY   Chopped and pounded stalks add flavor to fish, poultry sauces and stir-fries. The leaves are used in chicken and seafood dishes, curries, marinades, casseroles, soups, and stews. The leaves and stalks can be used after freezing, dried or fresh in all culinary endeavors.

MEDICINAL   Lemon Grass is an excellent insect repellent and is also used as a fungicide. Rub it on your skin to repel insects, or use it in a tea to help relieve congestion, coughing, bladder disorders, grouchiness, weariness, as a diuretic and sedative, or to help with headaches, fever, stomach aches, digestive problems, diarrhea, gas, bowel spasms, vomiting, flu symptoms, and as a mild sedative to promote perspiration. You can also convert Lemon Grass into an oil or capsule to use in place of a tea. Externally, Lemon Grass can be applied at a rate of ten drops of oil for athlete's foot, cuts, scrapes, where lower back pain occurs, to help with sciatica, sprains, tendonitis, neuralgia, circulation problems and rheumatism. It can help to clear up facial acne and clogged pores. For aromatherapy, add some leaves to a mesh bag and run under tap water for your bath, or simply cut some leaves and throw in the bath water for the same effect (or do both). A plant or two situated in a well-lighted window in the home will add a nice fragrance to the house. It is Not Recommended that Lemon Grass be used by young children, pregnant women and people with kidney or liver diseases.

More recently, Lemon Grass has been used as an additive in hair and soap products.

MYSTICAL   Lemon Grass is said to repel dragons and serpents. Burn it, bathe in it, or carry it on one's person for lust, fidelity, honesty, growth, strength, psychic powers, purification, and divination. Wear it as a charm, or in a sachet, to attract the object of your desire, and to bring honesty to your relationships. Add Lemon Grass leaves and stalks to your bath water to attract, and keep, a lover.

MARIJUANA

Cannabis spp.

Family	Cannabaceae – Hemp family
Origin	Central and southeast Asia
Zones	All
Type	Annual
Inclination	Non-invasive
Exposure	Full to half-sun
Start	Cuttings or seeds
Growth	To 6' x 3' on average
Flowers	Small, pale green
Harvest	Flowers and leaves
Fertilizer	Organic
Soil	Rich in organic material and well-drained
Tolerance	Keep on moist side
Attracts	Bees and butterflies
Seaside	Yes; requires protection from wind
Containers	Yes

USES

CULINARY   Today Marijuana is used in about every culinary dish imaginable as an additive. It can be prepared with cookies, cakes, pancakes, lasagna, macaroni, added to salads, etc.

MEDICINAL   Medical Marijuana is used in easing nausea and vomiting along with treating spasticity, painful conditions, muscular disorders (multiple sclerosis), asthma and glaucoma as well as allergies, inflammations, infections, epilepsy, depression, bipolar disorder, and anxiety disorder along with other maladies.

MYSTICAL   Among other things, it is said Marijuana can be burned as an incense to help promote body cleansing, for protection against evil and for calming effects.

MARJORAM

Origanum marjorana

Family	Lamiaceae – Mint family
Origin	North Africa, southeast Asia, the Mediterranean region, and Turkey
Zones	8-24
Type	Perennial – Marjoram should be treated as a summer annual in zones other than those listed above
Inclination	Non-invasive
Exposure	Full to half-sun
Start	Seeds in spring or early summer
Growth	To 2' x 2'
Flowers	Inconspicuous, small, and white; fragrant
Harvest	Leaves before flowering
Fertilizer	Organic
Soil	Rich, well drained
Tolerance	Average water; deer resistant
Attracts	Bees and butterflies
Seaside	Yes
Containers	Yes

USES

CULINARY Sweet Marjoram has been called a "chef's delight." It is used in much the same way as oregano and is of the same genus. Use it to flavor beef, veal, lamb, poultry, vegetables, potatoes, and stuffing. Use in marinades for artichoke hearts, asparagus, and mushrooms as well as in herb vinegars, oils, and butters.

MEDICINAL Use a Marjoram tea for relief from hay fever, sinus congestion, indigestion, asthma, stomach pain, headache, dizziness, colds, and nervous disorders. Use the tea unsweetened as a mouthwash or gargle. Grind Marjoram leaves into a paste and use for rheumatism and sprains or use a few drops of Marjoram oil for relief of toothache pain. Place in a cheese cloth under running bathwater as the leaves are believed to be mildly antiseptic and good for the skin.

MYSTICAL The ancient Greeks attributed Marjoram to the goddess of love (Aphrodite), therefore, it is considered one of the "love" herbs and has been used at wedding ceremonies down through the centuries. Legend has it that it you anoint yourself with Marjoram before bed you will dream of your future spouse. Place Marjoram around every room of your house for protection from negativity and evil intent. Mix it with violets when doing this to protect your family from colds and flu. Drink Marjoram tea for happiness, healing, love, money, health, peace, sleep, joy, good wishes, protection, and psychic enhancement. Put some in a mesh bag in bath water for love and peace. Burn it for help in accepting life changes, and for anti-sorcery spells. Carrying Marjoram in a sachet is said to help protect against evil and, added to food you share with the object of your affection, will strengthen your love for each other. Floral wreaths were worn by couples at both Greek and Roman marriages to symbolize the joyfulness of the wedding, and the happiness of the couple.

MINT

Mentha spp.

Family	Lamiaceae – Mint family
Origin	Asia and Europe
Zones	Zones vary but most mints grow anywhere
Type	Herbaceous perennial
Inclination	Invasive
Exposure	Sun or shade; does best in partial shade in hotter locations
Start	Cuttings in spring and summer, divisions anytime, or seeds in spring and summer
Growth	Growth rate varies by species, but most mints are generally regarded as groundcovers
Flowers	White to pale blue
Harvest	Leaves, best when young
Fertilizer	Not particular; pellet fertilizers can burn runners
Soil	Best in rich, well-drained soil
Tolerance	Drought tolerant once established; prefers moist soils but can grow under boggy conditions; deer resistant
Attracts	Bees and butterflies
Seaside	Yes
Containers	Yes

USES

CULINARY

Plants classified as Mints are some of the most widely used, flavorful and versatile herbs around. To name a few there are pineapple mint, chocolate, apple, licorice, lemon, orange, spearmint, peppermint, and pennyroyal to name a few. Mints are important commercially as flavorings and a source of menthol. All mints can be used in candies, cakes, cookies, etc. and are great in teas and to garnish fruit drinks. Some Mints, like peppermint, are stronger than others and may be too potent for home use but some, such as spearmint, compliment many dishes, including meat, fish, vegetables, soups, and sauces. Mints can also be used for adding flavor to fruit salads, cream, and cottage cheeses. Make your favorite tea and add a few leaves of your favorite Mint for a refreshing drink. Growing all the different Mints can give you a different flavored tea almost every day.

Modern day uses include Mints being used in cosmetics, perfumes, liniments, and cigarettes as well as breath fresheners, mouth rinses, toothpastes and chewing gum, and are being used extensively in aromatherapy. Powdered leaves help to whiten teeth.

MEDICINAL

Mints have it all and are an excellent source for reducing symptoms related to indigestion, stomach cramps, menstrual cramps, flatulence, upset stomach, vomiting, nausea as well as colic in children. Evidence of late hints that Mints may be useful in reducing the pain of arthritis and chronic joint pain. Use Mint oil on a cold compress or rub directly into the skin. Mint is also purported to repel insects, including mosquitoes.

MYSTICAL

In magic, Mints are premier healing herbs and can be used in incenses, healing charms, sachets and baths. Sprinkle Mint tea around the house for peace after an argument; drink Mint tea for its healing and calming properties before meditation or rituals. Place Mint leaves under, or in, the pillowcase for prophetic dreams. Carry the leaves in your wallet or purse to attract money and prosperity. In Greek Mythology, Mints were known as the "herbs of hospitality" and often used as room deodorizers. Today mints are used in cosmetics, perfumes, liniments and cigarettes as well as breath fresheners, mouth rinses, toothpastes and chewing gum, and are being used extensively in aromatherapy. Powdered leaves help whiten teeth.

OREGANO

Origanum vulgare

Family	Lamiacea – Mint family
Origin	Temperate Asia and Europe
Zones	1-24
Type	Perennial
Inclination	Non-invasive
Exposure	Full to half-sun with part shade in hotter locations
Start	Cuttings in spring and summer, divisions anytime, or seeds in spring; plants grown from seeds vary widely, so it is best to use divisions, or cuttings, from plants with flavors, and aromas, that suit you; for best leaf flavor keep plants from flowering
Growth	To 2' x 3'
Flowers	Varies; Rose-Pink, White, Purple and Purple-Pink
Harvest	Leaves
Fertilizer	Organic
Soil	Well-drained
Tolerance	Average water; becomes drought tolerant once established; deer resistant
Attracts	Bees and butterflies
Seaside	Yes; requires protection from wind
Containers	Yes

USES

CULINARY Like the other mints, Oregano has many and varied uses. There are many varieties of Oregano, so pick the ones you like for flavor, aroma, flowers, and foliage. Greek Oregano, perhaps the most popular of this species, can be used to flavor any culinary recipe or dish including pizza, pasta, many tomato-based dishes, and different Italian and Mexican sauces. Oregano can also be used in salads, stews, onion dishes and spaghetti, on roasts, poultry, game, shellfish, and olive oil along with vegetables, potatoes, cheese, and egg combination dishes. Just about anything you want to use it for will work.

MEDICINAL An Oregano herbal remedy can be used to treat urinary problems, headaches, swollen glands, flatulence, coughs, bronchitis, asthma, tonsillitis, menstrual problems, fevers, diarrhea, vomiting and jaundice. An oil is effective against toothaches and joint pains, as well as rheumatism, swelling, itching, aching muscles and sores. An unsweetened tea is useful as a gargle and mouthwash. Oregano can be used to help soothe your aches and pains by putting leaves in a mesh bag, and running beneath hot water, for your bath.

MYSTICAL To the ancient Greeks, Oregano reseeding itself on someone's grave signified that the happiness of the deceased person would be assured in the afterlife. As an off shoot, Oregano has become known as the herb of happiness, tranquility, good luck, health, protection and as help for the soul when having to let go of someone you love. Make a tea, or burn as an incense, to bring forth these magical powers. Plant around your house for protection and scatter inside, along with violets, to protect you and your family from colds. Carry Oregano around with you, in a sachet or charm, to bring good health and good luck, and wear it on your head, during sleep, to protect you and promote psychic dreams.

PARSLEY

Petroselinum crispum (curly leaf) and *P. neapolitanum* (flat leaf)

Family	Apiaceae – Parsley family
Origin	Western Asia and southern Europe
Zones	A3, 1-24
Type	Biennial, but usually grown as an annual
Inclination	Non-invasive; however, may self-sow under proper conditions
Exposure	Full to half-sun
Start	Seeds in early spring; best results for parsley is to start fresh each year by soaking seeds in warm water for 24 hours, before planting, to help germination as seeds are slow to start
Growth	Flat leaf to 2'-3' x 2', curly leaf to 6"-12" and as wide
Flowers	Inconspicuous, greenish white
Harvest	Leaves anytime, seeds when mature
Fertilizer	Organic
Soil	Rich, well-drained
Tolerance	Average water; becomes drought tolerant once established; deer resistant
Attracts	Bees
Seaside	Yes; requires protection from wind
Containers	Yes

USES

CULINARY Parsley is a familiar herb, and its usage is documented back to over 2,000 years ago. It is best known for its contribution to Italian cooking in dishes such as spaghetti and pizza. The flat-leaf variety is considered as having the best flavor in cooking, while the curly leafed varieties are used primarily as a garnish. Parsley is often used with roasted and stewed beef, in soups and stuffing's, with poultry, game, marinated vegetables, potatoes, cheese and egg combinations, onion dishes, shellfish and bell peppers. Parsley leaves can be used both fresh and dried.

MEDICINAL Parsley is considered a nutritional powerhouse. Since it contains a good deal of chlorophyll, it's considered a natural breath sweetener. Down through the centuries, Parsley tea has been used for kidney stones, bladder infections, jaundice, and enhanced digestion. Parsley is also regarded as an antispasmodic and to help relieve flatulence, while a tea made from the leaves and seeds are useful against dropsy, asthma, coughs and suppressed or difficult menstruation. Externally, an oil made of Parsley leaves and roots will repel head lice, and, as an ointment to ease joint pain and swellings. As a paste, Parsley is used to ease symptoms from bug bites and stings. Pick some leaves and squeeze the juice onto the bite for instant relief. Dip a cloth in unsweetened tea and place it over your closed eyes for about ten minutes to reduce fatigue and swelling of the eyes. Parsley is also used as a diuretic, and for gout and arthritis. Today oil derived from Parsley is used in commercial shampoos, soaps, perfumes, and skin lotions.

MYSTICAL The ancient Greeks used Parsley at funerals and wore the leaves and stems as wreaths long before this plant was recognized as a food. Corpses were sprinkled with the leaves to deodorize them. Parsley is associated with good luck, communicating with other planes, lust, protection, purification, fertility, reincarnation, health, strength, vitality, divination, passion, meditation, happiness, and rituals for the dead. A sprig of Parsley with your meal is supposed to protect you from contaminated food. Last, but not least, chewing on Parsley leaves is supposed to cover the smell of alcohol on your breath, so put it to beneficial use as a breath freshener when the cops pull you over.

PLANTAIN (RIBWORT)

Plantago lanceolata

Family	Plantaginaceae – Plantain family
Origin	Europe
Zones	All
Type	Perennial
Inclination	Invasive
Exposure	Full to half-sun
Start	Seeds in spring and summer
Growth	To 2' x 2'
Flowers	Inconspicuous, with greenish yellow color on stalks
Harvest	Leaves and seeds
Fertilizer	Any
Soil	Not particular but prefers rich and well-drained
Tolerance	Regular water
Attracts	Bees, birds, and butterflies
Seaside	No
Containers	Yes; recommended to keep plants under control

USES

CULINARY Plantain has no known culinary uses, but it is included in this book because of its considerable medicinal value. Considered an invasive weed, under cultivation it can become a welcome addition to the medicine cabinet.

MEDICINAL Plantain is a virtual medicinal cornucopia. Used externally it is effective when made into an ointment, or an oil, for helping to heal wounds, cuts, swelling, sprains, rashes, bruises, eczema, poison ivy, insect bites, diaper rash, hemorrhoids, boils, and blisters. It is also effective in drawing out bee sting poison, snakebite venom, and spider bites, and can be used to draw out thorns and splinters. Placed in shoes the leaves can help prevent blisters. Used as a tea, Plantain works well as a remedy for colds, flu, asthma, bronchitis, colic, emphysema, fevers, rheumatism, bladder problems, gastritis, hypertension, ulcers, irritable bowel syndrome, kidney stones, cystitis, sinusitis, goiter, PMS, diarrhea, hay fever, congestion, regulating menstrual flow, hoarseness and helps to stabilize blood sugar in diabetics. As a water infusion, the dried seeds can be used as a soothing eyewash, as a laxative, and for intestinal worms in children. It helps reduce prostatic swellings and again, taken as a tea, is a general detoxifier and has been reported, in this context, to help people quit smoking. Noted for its "body purifying" powers, Plantain cleans the system of heat, congestion, and toxic elements. The gum-like sap released by the plant offers comfort in case of physical disorders, particularly in the digestive, urinary and respiratory systems. Along with all the above, *P. amtaom* is used for tuberculosis, bowel, and stomach hemorrhaging, vomiting blood and is helpful in treating ear and urethra infections.

MYSTICAL Taken as a tea, Plantain is said to be useful for vivid dreams and divination as well as a protective herb when placed in a charm around a child's neck. For healing wishes, throw some dried leaves into a candle's flame, or into and an easterly wind. To increase the magical powers of other herbs, burn Plantain leaves and roots along with them.

ROSEMARY

Rosemarinus officinalis

Family	Lamiaceae – Mint family
Origin	Mediterranean
Zones	4-2, h1, h2; some varieties are hardier than others
Type	Evergreen perennial
Inclination	Non-invasive; however, may self-sow under proper conditions
Exposure	Full to ½ sun
Start	Cuttings, layering or seeds
Growth	Prostrate forms to 1' x 4'; upright to 6' x 4'
Flowers	Various shades of blue; occasionally white or pink; fragrant
Harvest	Leaves and flowers anytime
Fertilizer	Organic
Soil	Well-drained
Tolerance	Drought tolerant once established
Attracts	Bees, birds, and butterflies
Seaside	Yes – one of the best plants for windy, sea-salt sprayed places
Containers	Yes

USES

CULINARY — Rosemary is time-tested and one of the most popular herbs used for cooking purposes. It goes well with meat or fish, especially when roasted, and can be used to flavor tomato and other sauces. Rosemary also enhances cheeses, eggs, and vegetables along with thyme, bay, parsley, and chervil.

MEDICINAL — Rosemary is useful as a digestive aid, to treat headaches and muscle spasms, to reduce stress, as an expectorant, to help increase menstrual and urine flow and as a stimulant for the production of bile. Taken internally, Rosemary can irritate digestive organs so use sparingly. Make a tea to help relieve cold symptoms and as a beverage to help with headaches and low moods.

An infusion of Rosemary mixed with borax is said to produce a nice smelling hair wash used to help prevent dandruff and stimulate hair growth. This plant is also used to add fragrance to soaps and cosmetics.

MYSTICAL — Rosemary is believed to help with memory and learning. Put a sprig in your pocket, or a necklace around your neck, before a meeting, or other important situation, where mental clarity is important. Made into a wreath and placed above a door Rosemary is said to ward off evil. Putting a sprig under your pillow, or in your pillow case, will help ward off bad dreams. Place some Rosemary in cheesecloth, or a coffee filter, and place it under running bath water as a cleansing and purifying agent or use it to wash your hands before performing rituals. In Medieval times, Rosemary was associated with friendship, love and remembrance at weddings and funerals. Used in potpourri or sachets, Rosemary's fragrance is said to be of benefit in association with emotional spirit, pleasant memories and to help maintain a useful outlook on life.

SAGE – CULINARY

Salvia officinalis

Family	Lamiaceae – Mint family
Origin	Mediterranean coast and Spain
Zones	2-24, h1, h2
Type	Evergreen perennial
Inclination	Non-invasive
Exposure	Full to half-sun
Start	Cuttings, divisions, or seeds
Growth	To 3' x 2'
Flowers	Blue is most common; also comes in red, violet, red-violet, pink and white; fragrant
Harvest	Leaves anytime
Fertilizer	Organic
Soil	Average, well-drained
Tolerance	Drought tolerant once established; do not overwater
Attracts	Bees and butterflies
Seaside	Yes
Containers	Yes

USES

CULINARY There are over 100 varieties of Sage currently offered for sale on the market. Although many have culinary properties, *Salvia officinalis* is regarded by most as the "official" culinary and medicinal Sage. This popular plant is used to flavor meat, fish, stuffing's, salads, and soups, as well as enhancing bland vegetables such as potatoes, eggplant, and cheeses.

MEDICINAL This variety of Sage is widely used as an astringent and an antiseptic. As an antiseptic, it can be used in a tea to treat mouth sores, mouth ulcers, respiratory infections, congestion, coughs, sore throats, and to aid in the elimination of indigestion, fevers, night sweats, urinary problems, and is often used as an appetite stimulant. Sage has moisture drying properties and can be used as an antiperspirant. Its leaves can be used as a compress on cuts and wounds, and clinical studies show it can lower blood sugar in cases of diabetes. Sage has been used as an astringent in after shave lotion, and an infusion is said to color silver hair. Sage is sometimes used in a tea to help with flatulence and digestive problems. More recent studies have shown that Sage may play a key role in improving memory and in treating Alzheimer's disease. Because of its strength, using Sage is not recommended during pregnancy.

MYSTICAL Sage has long been burned to purify and cleanse a room of negative energy. In the 10th Century, Arab physicians said that Sage brought about a long and healthy life, and imported immortality. The Greeks and Romans believed that the smoke from burning Sage imparted wisdom and mental acuity. Carry some leaves of this plant in your wallet or purse to promote financial gain. Make a wish and write it on a leaf, and then hide it beneath your pillow. If you dream about your wish for three consecutive nights, your dream will come true. Burning Sage smells remarkably like burning marijuana, so keep that in mind if you have nosy neighbors.

SAINT JOHN'S WORT

Hypericum perforatum

Family	Hyperiaceae – St. John's Wort family
Origin	Asia and Europe
Zones	Vary by variety
Type	Perennial evergreen, semi-evergreen or deciduous, depending on variety and zone
Inclination	Generally non-invasive, except for the groundcover H. calycinum
Exposure	Full to half-sun; part shade in hotter climates
Start	Cuttings, clumps, or seeds
Growth	Varies by species; from 6" to 6' in height and 2' to 6' in width
Flowers	Yellow
Harvest	Leaves
Fertilizer	Organic
Soil	Does well in moist soils
Tolerance	All species do especially well in mild, moist regions
Attracts	Bees
Seaside	Yes
Containers	Yes

USES

CULINARY While St. John's Wort has little culinary use, it is included here because of its wide medicinal value, most recently believed to be a worthwhile agent when combating depression.

MEDICINAL Made into an ointment St. John's Wort can be applied to bruises, burns, wounds, hemorrhoids, sunburns, herpes sores, varicose veins, nerve pain and sciatica. An oil can be used for arthritis and rheumatism. Massaged around the spinal cord it is said to relieve back pain. As a tea, St. John's Wort is believed to relieve symptoms of anxiety, coughs, digestion, diarrhea, bronchial problems, depression, fatigue, flu, gout, insomnia, irritability, ulcers, and menstrual problems. Studies have shown that this plant may interfere with HIV and immune suppressants used in transplant patients, causing spikes in blood pressure in some people; therefore, consult your physician before use.

MYSTICAL St. John's Wort has long been associated with magic, and for centuries people thought that burning it would drive away evil spirits and demons. Somehow it became associated with Christianity and St. John the Baptist, from where it got its name. When carried in your wallet or purse, or elsewhere, it is believed to impart courage, protection, detecting other magicians, and strength when confronted with bad situations. Leaves made into a necklace are purported to ward off sickness and tension, and to enhance endurance and will during combat. Place sprigs of St. John's Wort in a jar on a windowsill for protection from lightening, fires, storms, and evil spirits. If you are a single woman, placing St. John's Wort under your pillow is said to induce dreams of your future husband.

SAVORY – SUMMER

Satureja hortensis

Family	Lamiaceae – Mint family
Origin	Southeastern Europe
Zones	All
Type	Annual
Inclination	Non-invasive
Exposure	Full sun best except in hottest climates
Start	Seeds
Growth	To 1 ½' x 1'
Flowers	Pinkish white to rose
Harvest	Flowers and leaves anytime
Fertilizer	Organic
Soil	Well-drained, but prefers organically enriched soil
Tolerance	Average water; prefers to be on dry side once established
Attracts	Bees and butterflies
Seaside	Not recommended
Containers	Yes

USES

CULINARY Summer Savory has been used to enhance foods for over 2,000 years. This annual variety is used to flavor soups, stews, liver, fish, butters, vinegars, peas, beans, eggs, meats, and many other vegetables as well as salads and stuffing's.

MEDICINAL As a tea, Summer Savory is said to help alleviate colic, diarrhea, flatulence, upset stomachs, mild sore throats, indigestion, and acts as an appetite stimulant as well as an expectorant. It has been used by diabetics, in a tea, to help with excessive thirst. A sprig of Summer Savory applied to wasp or bee stings provides instant relief. An ointment helps with minor rashes and skin irritations. The use of this plant is said to increase sex drive, while Winter Savory is said to decrease it.

MYSTICAL Carrying, burning, or eating Summer Savory will enhance your intellect, creativity and help you to enjoy a good life. The plant is said to attract males, happiness, and love. The word "Satyr," a mythical half-man, half-goat creature, is supposed to be a derivative of Satureja, who cultivated the plant to help people enjoy sex, drinks, and loud parties. To this day, Summer Savory is still believed to have aphrodisiac properties.

SAVORY – WINTER

Satureja montana

Family	Lamiaceae – Mint family
Origin	Southern Europe
Zones	3-11, 14-24
Type	Evergreen perennial
Inclination	Non-invasive
Exposure	Part sun
Start	Cuttings or seeds
Growth	To 15" x 2'
Flowers	Small, white to lilac whorls; fragrant
Harvest	Leaves anytime
Fertilizer	Organic
Soil	Light, well-drained
Tolerance	Average water
Attracts	Bees and butterflies
Seaside	Not recommended
Containers	Yes

USES

CULINARY   The main differences between Winter and Summer Savory are that the Winter variety is a perennial, and the summer variety is an annual. Also, Winter Savory has a stronger, more resinous flavor. Use Winter Savory to marinate meats, fish, vegetables, stuffing's, and egg dishes. Winter Savory is a great herb to use with bean dishes as it helps reduce gas associated with beans.

MEDICINAL   Winter Savory is used as an aid for intestinal disorders including cramps, indigestion, diarrhea, nausea, and intestinal gas. Like Summer Savory, the Winter variety is also used to treat coughs and sore throats, and to take the bite out of insect stings, including wasps and bees. Unlike Summer Savory, which is said to have aphrodisiac properties, Winter Savory is said to reduce sex drive.

MYSTICAL   The use of this plant has been associated with increased mental powers, happiness, laughter, and motivation.

SELF-HEAL (ALL-HEAL)

Prunella vulgaris

Family	Lamiaceae – Mint family
Origin	North Africa, America, Asia, and Europe
Zones	2-24
Type	Perennial
Inclination	Invasive
Exposure	Full sun to light shade
Start	Clumps or seeds
Growth	To 6" x 3'; usually used as a groundcover
Flowers	Light to dark pink, white and purple
Harvest	Leaves and stems
Fertilizer	Organic
Soil	Any
Tolerance	Prefers moist locations but becomes drought tolerant once established
Attracts	Bees and butterflies
Seaside	Yes
Containers	Yes

USES

CULINARY Self-Heal (Prunella) leaves are mildly bitter and can be used as salad greens or in soups, stews or boiled. A cold-water infusion of freshly chopped, or dried and powdered, leaves is a tasty and refreshing beverage.

MEDICINAL The common names "Self-Heal" and "All Heal" derive from use of the species to treat a large range of minor disorders. Prunella is reported to be useful for its antiseptic and antibacterial effects, and to help in cases of food poisoning, high blood pressure, cuts, and inflammations. While most of the uses are clinically untested, this plant has been shown to be an antioxidant, immune system stimulant, viral inhibitor, and an anti-inflammatory agent. A weak infusion is said to be excellent as an eye wash for pink eye. Taken internally as a medicinal tea, it is useful in the treatment of fevers, diarrhea, sore mouth and throat, internal bleeding along with weaknesses of the liver and heart. Made into a poultice, Self-Heal promotes healing of wounds and insect bites. Many Native American tribes used this plant for both food and medicine.

MYSTICAL Self-Heal was said to drive away the devil in medieval times, which led to the belief that the plant was grown in witch's gardens for just that purpose. Some Native American tribes used the roots to sharpen their powers of observation before going hunting.

TARRAGON, FRENCH

Artemesia dracunculus

Family	Asteraceae – Aster family
Origin	Caspian Sea region and Siberia
Zones	A1, a3, 2-10, 14-24
Type	Herbaceous perennial
Inclination	Non-invasive
Exposure	Full to half-sun
Start	Cuttings, divisions, or seeds
Growth	To 2' x 4'
Flowers	Inconspicuous, white flowers; leaves are aromatic when crushed
Harvest	Leaves
Fertilizer	Organic
Soil	Well-drained; mulch heavily in fall to help winter over
Tolerance	Average water; drought tolerant once established
Attracts	Bees
Seaside	Yes; requires protection from wind
Containers	Yes

USES

CULINARY Considered by many as the "King" of herbs, French Tarragon is a much-used herb in culinary circles and has an anise-like flavor. Along with flavoring sauces, butters, vinegars, soups, sour creams, and yogurt, it enhances fish, meat, poultry, game, eggs, lasagna and almost all mainstream vegetables. This plant is a main component of Béarnaise sauce.

MEDICINAL When mixed with Lemon Balm in a tea, it has been said to be effective for the prevention of the flu and herpes. French Tarragon is also effective for eliminating intestinal worms in children. As a tea it can be used for menstrual cramps, hyperactivity, depression, insomnia, stomach cramps, digestive problems, nerves, fatigue, and to increase appetite. French Tarragon has the unusual property of slightly numbing the mouth when the leaves are chewed and is therefore an effective remedy for dulling toothaches and cold sores. It is often used as a salt replacement for people on salt-restricted diets. Externally, French Tarragon leaves are helpful in relieving the symptoms of minor skin rashes and irritations.

MYSTICAL In Medieval times French Tarragon was believed to cure snakebite because of its serpentine root system. It is considered a protective and calming herb. In the kitchen its powers are said to put guests at ease and to make them feel welcome. Carried as a charm, or in sachets, it will bring compassion, love, peace, good luck, and nurturing. Used as incense it is considered a banishing herb. Write down what it is you want to banish, on a white piece of paper, and then burn the paper over the incense.

TARRAGON, MEXICAN

Tagetes lucida

Family	Asteraceae – Marigold family
Origin	Mexico and southwestern United States
Zones	8-10, 12-24
Type	Perennial
Inclination	Non-invasive
Exposure	Full to half-sun
Start	Cuttings or seeds
Growth	To 3' x 3'
Flowers	Yellow-gold
Harvest	Leaves
Fertilizer	Organic
Soil	Average
Tolerance	Average water; drought tolerant once established
Attracts	Bees
Seaside	Yes
Containers	Yes

USES

CULINARY — Although not related to French Tarragon, this plant has similar properties for culinary use and can be used as a substitute for the French variety when it is unavailable, or if you wish to use a spicier version of Tarragon. Because of its spicy nature Mexican Tarragon is a favorite ingredient in Mexican and southwestern United States cuisine. The leaves of this plant are often used as a garnish as well as a flavoring in butter, and on poultry.

MEDICINAL — Used in a tea, Mexican Tarragon has been used as an aphrodisiac in Mexico since colonial times. Internally it is useful in fighting nausea, diarrhea, indigestion, colic, hiccups, malaria, and fevers. Externally Mexican Tarragon is used to treat scorpion bites and to remove ticks. Burning dried leaves is said to repel insects. It is also purported to calm upset stomachs, soothe frayed nerves, and treat hangovers. In India, juice from the leaves is used to treat eczema.

MYSTICAL — Being an American Continent native plant there is not much history concerning this variety of Tarragon; however, it is said that the Aztecs used it as an incense in rituals and to treat people stricken by lightning. Also, its leaves were an important flavoring in "Chocolati," a foaming, cocoa based drink of the Aztecs, and it was sprinkled on the faces of prisoners of war so they would be sedated when they were burned as sacrifices.

THYME

Thymus vulgaris

Family	Lamiacea – Mint family
Origin	Mediterranean
Zones	1-24
Type	Evergreen perennial
Inclination	Non-invasive
Exposure	Full to half-sun, light shade in hotter climates
Start	Cuttings in summer, root divisions or seeds
Growth	To 1' x 2'; classified as groundcover
Flowers	White to lilac in late spring and summer
Harvest	Leaves anytime
Fertilizer	Organic
Soil	Light and well-drained
Tolerance	Some drought tolerance when established
Attracts	Bees
Seaside	Yes
Containers	Yes

USES

CULINARY — There are many varieties of Thyme in cultivation, but this is the most common one used for culinary purposes. "When in doubt, use Thyme" is a favorite saying among cooks. It is used as a garnish in salads and chowders. Use dried or fresh leaves for seasoning fish, shellfish, poultry stuffing, soups, and vegetables.

MEDICINAL — During Medieval times, Thyme was prescribed for epilepsy and melancholy. Nowadays, it has been used to treat intestinal worms, bronchial and gastrointestinal ailments, laryngitis, diarrhea, and loss of appetite. Thyme is also an antiseptic and can be used as a skin cleanser, is effective against fungi and bacteria, helps in eradicating lice, scabies and crabs and helps relieve urinary infections, nervous depression as well as improve liver function, and provide relief for bruises and sprains.

MYSTICAL — Place fresh sprigs of Thyme in a pillow to promote sleep and prevent nightmares. As an incense it is thought to enhance psychic powers and renew energy. Burning it in the home will banish evil and purify the home. Carry it on your person to promote courage, good health and protect from negativity. Used in a bath it is said to remove sorrows and ills from the past. When drunk as a tea, in medieval times, it was said to have enabled people to see nymphs and fairies. During the same period, if knights received a sprig of Thyme from their ladies, it was said to keep up their spirits when going into battle.

VALERIAN (GARDEN HELIOTROPE)

Valeriana officinalis

Family	Valerianaceae– Valerian family
Origin	Western Asia and Europe
Zones	1-24
Type	Perennial
Inclination	Invasive; roots attract cats in similar fashion to catnip
Exposure	Full to half-sun
Start	Divisions or seeds
Growth	To 5' x 2'
Flowers	Pink, red or white and have a cherry-pie fragrance; however, leaves have an unfavorable smell; flowers were used in perfumes in the 16th century
Harvest	Roots
Fertilizer	Organic
Soil	Not particular
Tolerance	Average water
Attracts	Bees and butterflies
Seaside	Not recommended
Containers	No

USES

CULINARY   None known.

MEDICINAL   Valerian roots have been used as a sleeping aid for over 1,000 years without the side effects of grogginess in the morning, plus it does not interact with alcohol as prescription drugs do. Valerian can be dried and used in tea and capsules or distilled into oils and ointments. It has been used in cases of nervous tension, is an effective stress reducer, and helps with depression, hysteria, panic, irritability, anxiety, fear, stomach cramping, indigestion, delusions, exhaustion, and insomnia. Valerian is useful as a digestive aid and helps alleviate gas, diarrhea, and ulcer pain. Testing has shown that it also eases muscle cramping, rheumatic pain, migraines, uterine cramps, intestinal colic as well as stress-related heart problems and hypertension. Finally, it also has benefits in cases of sciatica, multiple sclerosis, shingles, epilepsy, and peripheral neuropathy to include numbness, tingling, muscle weakness, pain in the extremities and helps with asthma attacks. Valerian is not recommended for pregnant and breast-feeding women.

MYSTICAL   Valerian is said to offer protection, purification, consecration, love, and harmony when used with rituals and spells. For protection from evil, carry Valerian with you. Sachets placed around the home protect against lightning strikes and placed in your pillow protects against nightmares. A few leaves placed in your shoes protects against colds and flu. Leaves in the immediate vicinity help restore harmony to quarreling couples and growing the plant on your property ensures harmony with your spouse. Valerian can be used to purify ritual spaces and consecrate incense burners. Dried Valerian stalks can be soaked in tallow or oil, then used as a torch, improving clarity for a given situation.

VIOLET

Viola species

Family	Violacea – Violet family
Origin	North Africa, North America, Asia, Australia, and Europe
Zones	Zones vary; all species do well in cool and cold weather climates
Type	Annuals, perennials
Inclination	Most species reseed under proper conditions
Exposure	Full to half-sun or shade; shade to part shade in hotter climates
Start	Cuttings, divisions, or seeds
Growth	To around 8" x 1'; used primarily in borders and as a groundcover
Flowers	Blue, pink, purple, white, yellow, and multi-colored; fragrant
Harvest	Flowers and leaves anytime
Fertilizer	Organic
Soil	Prefers loamy soil
Tolerance	Keep moist for best results
Attracts	Bees and butterflies
Seaside	Yes
Containers	Yes

USES

CULINARY Leaves and flowers, which are tart and sweet, can be eaten alone or used in salads, on grilled meats, in soups, stews, stir-fries and in steamed vegetables. Flowers can be used as a festive touch in punches, and the petals candied and used to garnish cakes, fruits, and pastries. Make Violet water by steeping leaves and flowers until the mix becomes fragrant. You can then use the water in teas, puddings and for flavoring ice cubes.

MEDICINAL Teas and oils can be used to help treat bronchitis, coughs, colds, fevers, asthma, constipation, arthritis, sore throats, and tonsillitis. Teas can also be used as a gargle or made into syrup by adding honey and using for the same purpose. Use as a laxative, for insomnia and for reducing the symptoms of a hangover, neck pain and headache. As a paste, Violets are purported to relieve rheumatism. As an ointment, Violets are helpful in relieving various skin eruptions and sores.

MYSTICAL When mixed with Lavender in a sachet, Violets make a strong combination for love (they have been used in love potions) and are associated with dedication and loyalty. Carry Violets on your person for good luck and putting flowers in your pillow enhances prophetic dreams and divination. Use the leaves to absorb evil spells and ill will. If Violets appear in your dreams, your life will change for the better. If you harvest the first Violet of spring, your wish will be granted. Violets can also be used in spells for money, protection, good luck, faithfulness, lust, wishes, peace, and healing, and are especially useful after a relationship breaks up.

YARROW

Achillea millefolium

Family	Asteraceae – Aster family
Origin	Asia and Europe; naturalized in North America
Zones	A1-a3, 1-24
Type	Perennial
Inclination	Invasive if left unattended; will reseed under proper conditions
Exposure	Full to half-sun
Start	Divisions or seeds
Growth	Plants to 2' x 2', flower stalks to 3'
Flowers	Pink, red, yellow or white; achillea filipendulina has yellow flower stalks to 5'; fragrant
Harvest	Flowers and leaves
Fertilizer	Any
Soil	Not particular but prefers well-drained
Tolerance	Drought tolerant once established
Attracts	Bees, butterflies, and other beneficial insects
Seaside	Yes
Containers	Yes

USES

CULINARY — Used in herbal teas and beer. Can be used as a substitute for sage in recipes.

MEDICINAL — Taken internally, as a tea, Yarrow is believed to aid in digestion and increased appetite. Undocumented uses throughout history include relief from stomach cramps, kidney and urinary tract problems, rheumatism, menstrual cramping, hypertension, flatulence, toothaches, snake bites, nausea, and diarrhea. Externally, make a tea with the flower tops and use as an astringent for acne, skin tone and hair conditioner. Crush the leaves and use immediately to help stop bleeding of wounds, cuts, and scrapes, and to aid in the healing of rashes and burns. Use Yarrow in the bath to help soothe hemorrhoids. Yarrow should not be used by pregnant women.

MYSTICAL — When drunk as a tea Yarrow is believed to increase psychic power and powers of perception. When burned, if the smoke goes up, it is a good omen, if down. a bad one. Use Yarrow flowers in sachets for love and charms. If placed underneath a pillow before sleep, it will produce dreams of your lover. Hanging flowers over your bridal bed will insure love that lasts at least seven years. If you use Yarrow in spells and rituals it will draw the attention of long-lost friends and lovers. Carried in your hand Yarrow will ward off fear. Carried in your pocket or purse Yarrow reverses negativity and protects from hexes. Add to your bath to protect from evil and harm. Throwing Yarrow flowers across the threshold will protect your home from evil and, tied to an infant's cradle, will protect the child from harmful forces.

An Introduction to Native American Herbs

By the time European settlers began arriving in America there were over 2,000 fully established Native American tribes with sustainable medical practices. The "Medicine Man/Woman" was cared for and protected by those in their village and, in return, they took care of the physical and emotional health of the tribe. Many of the herbs utilized by the tribes were adopted by settlers, and eventually made their way back to Europe where many are still in use to this day. Unfortunately, as mentioned previously, due to a lack of a written language, many plants and their remedies were lost down through the ages but, as with the trend toward the more popular and well-known herbal medicines, many are making a comeback. They are included in this book because some of them may be growing in your own back yard where you might want to try them, perhaps as a means to defray the never ending, rising cost of prescription drugs, and as a way toward a healthier lifestyle.

WARNING!

This information is provided purely for historical and cultural purposes. Many herbs used by Native Americans have been omitted due to scanty information and a general lack of verifiability. If used improperly, as with any medicine, the herbs described herein can be dangerous, if not fatal. Never use any remedy without the advice of an herbalist, a professional cook, professional healthcare provider, your doctor, information derived from the internet, or perhaps your neighbor down the street who has used one or more of them with success over the years.

An Introduction to Native American Herbal Remedies

According to Native American folklore, the Creator, or Great Spirit, provided through Mother Nature, a cure for every ailment. Unfortunately, unlike our ancient European, Asian, and Middle Eastern ancestors, Native Americans never mastered the art of writing; therefore, the information obtained regarding Native American herbs has been passed down over the centuries primarily by word of mouth. Much of that was lost over the years once the European races began colonizing North America, exploiting Native Americans, and destroying their cultures in the process. Despite that, there are still many North American herbs that managed to get recorded before all knowledge of them vanished.

How did our Native Americans come to discover herbs? No one knows for sure, but it probably happened something like this: Starving, a young Indian mother scours the forests and meadows looking for something to eat, finally hitting upon a plant that doesn't kill her, or make her sick in the process of sampling it, and soon her tribe has a new source of food. Similarly, someone gets stung by a bee and, in desperation, grabs the leaf of some nearby plant and rubs it on the sting, feeling relief as the pain ebbs away. In Gaea and Shandor Weiss' book "Growing & Using Healing Herbs" (Rodale Press, 1985) Wallace Black Elk, a Sioux medicine man, states that his tribe learned the value of herbs by watching what plants deer and other animals ate, and then incorporating them into their diets. There are many ways our ancestors could have discovered herbs, through trial and error, and perhaps with lives lost along the way.

Medicine men and women were the healers of their tribes in days gone by, not only spiritually, but medicinally as well. There are many documented stories of the vast knowledge of herbs these Native American doctors used to help heal sickness in their camps. Yet again, unlike the old-world people, there was no written word of what they knew and, while the people of the tribes they prescribed for were well taken care of, these prescriptions were seldom passed from tribe to tribe so that, over time, what one group of Native Americans knew, another did not. Also, herbs are zone specific, which is to say most of them only grow in certain areas and thus were only able to be utilized by tribes indigenous to those areas. Despite these challenges an amazing amount of herbal wisdom has been accumulated over the years from the differing tribes living in North America. On the following pages you will find what herbs and plants our Native American ancestors used to help benefit the well-being of their brothers and sisters and, in modern times, the rest of us. Like the other herbs listed in this book there are no guarantees that the benefits they prescribe will work, but there's no proof they won't, either. That said, like all the herbs listed in this book, use them at your own risk.

Sources: The Cherokee Messenger by Judy Nolan; Native American Herbal Remedies www.herbsforhealth.about.com/cs/Amerindianherbs/; Natural Remedies Encyclopedia Millspaugh, Charles F.; American Medicinal Plants. NY: Dover Publications (1974); Mooney, James; Myths of the Cherokee and Sacred Formulas of the Cherokees. Nashville, TN: Charles and Randy Elders, Publishers, 1982; Weiner, Michael; Earth Medicine Earth Food, NY: Fawcett columbine, 1980.

ASPEN – QUAKING

Populus tremuloides

Family	Salicaceae – Willow family
Origin	North America
Zones	1-7
Type	Deciduous tree; aspens are the most widely distributed tree in North America
Inclination	Non-invasive
Exposure	Sun
Start	Cuttings, root divisions or seeds
Growth	To 50' x 25'; fast
Flowers	Catkins, generally small and white
Harvest	Bark and leaves
Fertilizer	Any
Soil	Not particular
Tolerance	Keep on moist side for best results
Attracts	Butterflies and moths
Seaside	Yes
Containers	Not recommended

USES

CULINARY North American Native's cut the inner bark into strips, dried the strips, and then ground them into a meal to be mixed with other grains for bread or mush. The catkins were eaten whole while the cambium layer was eaten raw or used in soups.

MEDICINAL The bark was used to treat fevers, scurvy, coughs, pain, and as an anti-inflammatory agent. Today, Quaking Aspen is used to relieve pain in rheumatic disorders including arthritis, back pain, bursitis, carpal tunnel syndrome, Crohn's Disease, inflammatory bowel disease, fibromyalgia, and tempo mandibular joint disorder.

MYSTICAL Modern legend has it that aspen buds, or leaves, carried on your person, will attract money.

BLACKBERRY, AMERICAN

Rubus ursinus

Family	Rosaceae – Rose family
Origin	Western and northwestern America
Zones	1-7
Type	Perennial woody vine
Inclination	Invasive, but not as invasive as European and Himalayan varieties
Exposure	Sun or part shade
Start	Cuttings, layering or seeds
Growth	10' to 20' in all directions
Flowers	White to pink, bloom in clusters
Harvest	Berries in fall, flowers in spring
Fertilizer	Not particular
Soil	Any, but prefers deep, well-drained soil
Tolerance	Prefers moist to wet conditions, but will die in standing water
Attracts	Bees
Seaside	Yes
Containers	No

Uses

Culinary Native Americans ate the ripened fruit when available. Blackberry fruit was dried with meat to make cakes, which were eaten in winter. Un-ripened, green berries were soaked in water to make a refreshing drink, and leaves were used in making teas.

Modern day uses include using American Blackberry in a variety of teas, jams, jellies, fruit drinks, pies, etc. The young shoots can be eaten raw or cooked like asparagus. Flowers are sometimes used in salads.

Medicinal A decoction of the vines and roots were used in the treatment of vomiting and the spitting of blood. A tea, made from blackberry roots, was used by Native Americans as a remedy for diarrhea and dysentery. Ripe berries were added to bitter medicines to sweeten them, while the thorny stems were used in scrubbing.

Mystical None known.

BLADDERPOD (FENDLER'S)

Lesquerella fendleri

Family	Brassicaceae – Mustard family
Origin	Southwestern United States
Zones	6-11
Type	Perennial shrub
Inclination	Non-invasive
Exposure	Part shade
Start	Seeds
Growth	To 16" x 8"
Flowers	Yellow flowers on 1' spikes
Harvest	Leaves
Fertilizer	Any
Soil	Well-drained
Tolerance	Drought tolerant once established
Attracts	Bees, birds, and butterflies
Seaside	Not recommended
Containers	Yes

USES

CULINARY None known.

MEDICINAL The Navajo made a tea from the plant and used it for spider bites. The crushed leaves of Bladderpod were also used for swellings, snake bites, toothaches, and sore eyes.

Fendler's Bladderpod is currently under study for use as a protein supplement in both human and animal food. The oil from the seeds can be used as a replacement for castor oil in some cases and is also used in high performance lubricants and as an additive in paints, plastics, pharmaceuticals, and cosmetics.

MYSTICAL None known.

BLOODROOT

Sanguinaria canadensis

Family	Papaveraceae – Poppy family
Origin	Eastern United States
Zones	3-9
Type	Perennial
Inclination	Non-invasive
Exposure	Semi-shade is best
Start	Root divisions or seeds
Growth	To 10" x 8"
Flowers	White with yellow centers
Harvest	Roots
Fertilizer	Compost or manure
Soil	Prefers soils rich in humus and well-drained
Tolerance	Always keep moist
Attracts	Bees and beetles
Seaside	Not recommended
Containers	Yes

USES

CULINARY None known.

MEDICINAL Among Native Americans of the Mississippi region, Bloodroot was a favorite rheumatism remedy, while the Rappahannock of Virginia drank a tea made from the roots for many ailments. The flowers and leaves were used to create insect repellents, sedatives, and tonics, as well as helping to relieve aching throats and cure cancers. A poultice was used to treat skin ulcers, warts, athlete's foot, other fungal conditions, and acute muscle pain.

Modern day uses of Bloodroot include promoting coughing to clear mucus, acting as a plaque inhibitor in toothpastes, treating fevers and rheumatism, ulcers, ringworm, and skin infections. Roots have been used to produce red, orange, and pink dyes.

MYSTICAL An old Cherokee myth states that a small piece of Bloodroot, carried in a medicine bag, would ward off evil spirits.

BLUE COHOSH

Caulophyllum thalictroides

Family	Berberidacea – Barberry family
Origin	Eastern United States
Zones	3-9
Type	Perennial
Inclination	Non-invasive
Exposure	Shade
Start	Divisions or seeds
Growth	To 3' x 3'
Flowers	Yellow-green to brown
Harvest	Roots and seeds
Fertilizer	Compost
Soil	Rich in organic matter
Tolerance	Keep moist
Attracts	Bees
Seaside	Yes; grow in protected areas
Containers	Yes

USES

CULINARY Roasted seeds can be used as a coffee substitute.

MEDICINAL Blue Cohosh is one of the more useful American plants for medicinal purposes. Some Native American tribes used an infusion of the roots in water, drunk over several weeks, to speed child birth, or to prevent conception. It was also used in treatments for arthritis, epilepsy, child colic, fits and hysterics, gallstones, fevers, hiccupping, sore throats and as a general, overall tonic. Chippewa women drank a strong decoction of powdered Blue Cohosh root to promote child birth and menstruation.

In more modern times Blue Cohosh is shown to have anti-inflammatory uses in the treatment of rheumatism and is also used for worms and parasites in the human gastrointestinal system. This plant induces child birth in various cultures throughout the modern world, cures uterine inflammations and is also an effective diuretic. Because of its unique properties it has also been used as an abortifacient.

MYSTICAL None known.

BONESET (FEVERWORT)

Eupatorium perfoliatum

Family	Asteraceae – Aster family
Origin	Eastern United States
Zones	2-10
Type	Perennial shrub
Inclination	Non-invasive
Exposure	Full to half-sun
Start	Cuttings, divisions, or seeds
Growth	To 3' x 3'
Flowers	White
Harvest	Leaves
Fertilizer	Organic
Soil	Sandy, loamy or clay
Tolerance	Keep moist
Attracts	Butterflies
Seaside	Yes; requires protection from wind
Containers	Yes

USES

CULINARY A refreshing tea can be made using dried Boneset leaves.

MEDICINAL Reduces or eliminates many problems associated with PMS, including irritability, depression, bloating, and breast pain. If taken regularly, Evening Primrose is purported to regulate menstrual periods and, in fact, in Europe, the oil is already established as an excellent remedy for PMS. Taken as a tea it helps fight obesity. Other problems for which the oil (taken internally) is used include asthma, cholesterol regulation, arteriosclerosis, prostate health, allergies, headaches, and rheumatoid arthritis, multiple sclerosis, lupus, and scleroderma. Also, the oil helps alleviate complications arising from diabetes including numbness, tingling and poor circulation as well as treating cirrhosis of the liver. Externally the leaves, stems, and roots, used as a tea, are nourishing for the skin, and is used in treatment of acne, dry skin, rashes, itchiness, eczema and for overall skin health. Eating the flowers, leaves, or roots, provides the same health benefits as taking commercial oil preparations. Native Americans used Evening Primrose to treat stomach aches, hemorrhoids, sore throats, and scrapes.

MYSTICAL Boneset tea was one of the most frequently used medicinal plants during past centuries. The Menominee used it to reduce fevers, while the Alabama used it to treat stomach aches. The Creek utilized Boneset to reduce body pain and the Iroquois and Mohegan for fevers and colds. It was also used to treat loss of appetite and indigestion. Boneset reduces fevers by encouraging sweating, loosening phlegm, and promoting its removal through coughing. The Cherokee drank a decoction of the herb to cure fevers, while early colonists considered it a "Cure All."

Boneset is considered to be among the most useful of Native American plants. Extracts are now used in herbal medicine for fevers, colds and influenza, bronchitis, pneumonia, and other ailments attributed to the common cold. Currently, herbalists also recommend Boneset for relieving aches and pains associated with fevers, coughing, congestion, arthritis, and rheumatism.

BROOM SNAKEWEED

Gutierrezia sarothrae

Family	Asteraceae – Sunflower family
Origin	Western North America
Zones	5-9
Type	Perennial shrub
Inclination	Can become invasive in some regions and habitats
Exposure	Sun
Start	Seeds
Growth	To 2' x 2'
Flowers	Golden yellow clusters at end of stems
Harvest	Seeds
Fertilizer	Not particular
Soil	Keep on dry side; does not like constantly moist or wet soil
Tolerance	Drought tolerant as it is a desert native
Attracts	Birds
Seaside	Not recommended
Containers	Yes

USES

CULINARY   The Hidatsa tribe of North America harvested the dried seeds from Broom Snakeweed, then mixed and ground them with corn, squash, and beans to make a seed ball to ward off hunger, sleep, and general weariness.

MEDICINAL   Broom Snakeweed was widely used by Native Americans for a variety of purposes. Comanche and other tribes used the plant stems to make brooms for sweeping their residences, thus the name "Broom." The Lakota used a decoction to treat colds, coughs, and dizziness. They, as well as the Mohawk, chewed the plant and applied it to wounds, snake bites and stings from insects. Navajo women drank a tea of the whole plant to promote the expulsion of the placenta. The Navajo sprinkled ashes over their bodies to treat headaches and dizziness, while the Blackfoot used the roots in an herbal steam for treatment of respiratory illnesses.

MYSTICAL   None known.

BUCKWHEAT, RED

Eriogonum grande rubescens

Family	Polygonaceae – Buckwheat family
Origin	Northwestern Baja California, California coastal areas and Channel Islands
Zones	8-10
Type	Perennial shrub
Inclination	Non-invasive
Exposure	Full to half-sun
Start	Seeds
Growth	To 1' x 3'
Flowers	Pink, red and white
Harvest	Seeds
Fertilizer	Not particular
Soil	Prefers dry clay
Tolerance	Drought tolerant
Attracts	Bees and butterflies
Seaside	Yes
Containers	Yes

USES

CULINARY	Edible seeds and shoots.
MEDICINAL	Hopi women were given an infusion of the entire Buckwheat plant to stop bleeding. The Cahuilla used the leaves closest to the roots as a cathartic, and, with an infusion of flowers, as an eyewash. Internally, Buckwheat was used to clean out the intestines and to shrink the uterus and reduce dysmenorrhea. The Hopi, Navajo and Kayenta used the plant as an analgesic for severe back and hip pain, especially in pregnant women. The Kawaiisu used a decoction of the roots for diarrhea and as a heart medicine. The Mahuna used an infusion of flowers and leaves as a mouthwash for pyorrhea. The Thompson used Buckwheat plants in steam baths for aching and rheumatic joints, as well as making a salve of leaf ashes, mixed with grease, for swellings. A decoction was taken for stomach pain and syphilis. The Cahuilla and Tubatulabal ate the seeds and shoots for food. Obviously, because Red Buckwheat grows naturally in only a few places, there was much trading between the coastal tribes and those situated farther inland (Hopi, Navajo) for this plant to be of so much use to so many tribes.
MYSTICAL	None known.

CHOKECHERRY

Prunus virginiana

Family	Rosaceae – Rose family
Origin	North America
Zones	3-8
Type	Perennial tree
Inclination	Invasive suckers
Exposure	Sun to part shade
Start	Cuttings or seeds
Growth	To 30' x 20'
Flowers	White in hanging clusters; fragrant
Harvest	Fruit in fall – Do not eat seeds or leaves
Fertilizer	All-purpose, compost, manure, fruit, and nut food
Soil	Prefers rich, moist soil; but does well in a wide range of soils, from sandy to clays that have a limestone base
Tolerance	Average water for best results; considered drought tolerant
Attracts	Bees, birds, butterflies, deer, and other wildlife; leaves and seeds are poisonous
Seaside	Yes; requires protected locations
Containers	Not recommended

USES

CULINARY	For many Native American tribes Chokecherries were one of the most important foods in their diets.
MEDICINAL	Native Americans used a concoction of Chokecherry roots and bark to ward off, or treat, colds, fevers, stomachaches, malaria, tuberculosis, and intestinal worms. A tea from the bark was used as a sedative.
MYSTICAL	In modern times the ripened fruit of the Chokecherry has been used to make jams, jellies, syrups, pies, wines, etc. Chokecherries are more astringent, and bitter, that its cousin the wild black cherry, requiring more work (and lots of sugar) to produce products similar to those made from the wild black cherry, *Prunus serotina*.

CREOSOTE BUSH

Larrea tridentata

Family	Zygophyllaceae – Creosote bush family
Origin	Southwestern United States deserts - a clone-colony creosote bush near Lucerne, California, is considered one of the oldest living organisms on earth at an estimated 11,700 years old!
Zones	8-10; okay in other zones if planted in sandy, well-drained soil
Type	Perennial shrub
Inclination	Non-invasive
Exposure	Full to half-sun
Start	Seeds after last frost; scarification is recommended as well as pouring hot water over seeds and letting them soak for 24 hours to help germination
Growth	To 6' x 6'; can reach 10' and larger under best conditions
Flowers	Yellow and fragrant; leaves are also fragrant after a rain
Harvest	Seeds
Fertilizer	Not particular
Soil	Sandy, well-drained
Tolerance	Drought tolerant
Attracts	Bees and deer
Seaside	Yes, in well-drained, sandy soil
Containers	Yes

USES

CULINARY   None known.

MEDICINAL   A tea made from the leaves was used by southwestern Native American tribes for bronchial and other respiratory problems, as well as helping to relieve constipation and menstrual cramps. Also, a powder made from dried leaves was used to fight infections when applied to cuts, burns and wounds. As a side note, a sticky substance, secreted by scale insects that infest the plant, was used to mend waterproof baskets and pottery.

MYSTICAL   None known.

DEVIL'S CLAW

Proboscidea parviflora

Family	Martynaceae – Unicorn plant family
Origin	Southwestern United States deserts
Zones	7-10
Type	Annual
Inclination	Non-invasive
Exposure	Full sun
Start	Seeds; soak in warm water eight hours before planting
Growth	To 2' x 4'
Flowers	Pink, purple or white
Harvest	Seeds
Fertilizer	All-purpose
Soil	Sandy, well-drained
Tolerance	Drought tolerant
Attracts	Bees
Seaside	Unknown
Containers	Yes

USES

CULINARY   The Papago tribe used the young seed pods for food while the Pima cracked the seeds between their teeth and ate them like pine nuts.

MEDICINAL   The Pima broke a small piece of the claw off and pressed it into the flesh, then lighted it and allowed it to burn to treat rheumatism. Today the dried "claws" that tip each fruit are used in baskets, weaved chairs, etc., to improve their durability.

MYSTICAL   Certain decorative patterns created by Devil's Claw fibers are considered sacred. The Papago believed the Great Spirit showed women how to weave Devil's Claw fibers into different patterns that were used to identify the baskets of each family or village.

DOGBANE (INDIAN HEMP)

Apocynum cannabinum

Family	Apocynaceae – Dogbane family
Origin	North America
Zones	1-10
Type	Perennial
Inclination	Invasive
Exposure	Full sun
Start	Cuttings, root divisions or seeds
Growth	To 6' x 4'
Flowers	White to greenish white
Harvest	Seeds and stems
Fertilizer	Not particular
Soil	Well-drained
Tolerates	Keep moist
Attracts	Butterflies, flies, and wasps
Seaside	Yes
Containers	Not recommended

USES

CULINARY Dogbane is considered highly toxic and can prove fatal if used incorrectly.

MEDICINAL The boiled roots of Dogbane were made into teas to treat syphilis, rheumatism, intestinal worms, asthma, dysentery, and fevers. It was used by the Potawatomi as a heart medicine, the fruit boiled while it was still green, and the resulting decoction drunk. It was also used for kidney problems, dropsy, as an oral contraceptive, to reduce high blood pressure and also used as a sedative and mild hypnotic.

Several Native American tribes used Dogbane fibers to make nets, fishing line fabric, twine, bow-strings and for sewing. Modern day uses include the manufacturing of paper, cordage, construction materials, textiles, clothing, biofuels, and medical products.

MYSTICAL A charm was made from the plant and used to ward off "bad medicine" and evil influences.

DOGWOOD, EASTERN

Cornus florida

Family	Cornaceae – Dogwood family
Origin	Eastern United States
Zones	5-9
Type	Deciduous small tree
Inclination	Non-invasive
Exposure	Shade to part shade
Start	Cuttings or seeds
Growth	To 30' x 30'
Flowers	White to pink
Harvest	Bark and seeds
Fertilizer	Compost, manure, and organics
Soil	Rich, moist and well-drained
Tolerance	Keep out of hot, direct sun
Attracts	Bees; berries attract birds
Seaside	Yes; requires protected location
Containers	Not recommended

USES

CULINARY Berries are edible but not tasty.

MEDICINAL The Menominee boiled the inner bark of the Dogwood and passed the warm solution into the rectum with a rectal syringe made from the bladder of a small mammal, along with the hollow bone of a bird, to alleviate pain. The bark was also boiled in water and the extract was utilized to ease sore and painful muscles. An herbal tea was prepared and used to induce perspiration to help cure fevers. Also, the Delaware boiled the inner bark in water making a tea to reduce fevers.

Eastern Dogwood was used in the past, and in some cases still is, to produce inks, scarlet dyes and as a quinine substitute. The dense wood has also been used for golf club heads, wooden rake teeth, tool handles, jeweler's boxes, and butcher's blocks among other things.

MYSTICAL In Native American lore an Indian princess, killed by a suitor she refused, used dogwood petals to dab blood from her wounds while she died. The myth says this act led to the Dogwood flowers' red markings on the petals.

EVENING PRIMROSE (SUN DROP)

Oenothera biennis

Family	Onagraceae – Evening Primrose family
Origin	North and South America
Zones	3-11
Type	Herbaceous biennial
Inclination	Can become invasive in some regions and habitats
Exposure	Full to half-sun
Start	Seeds
Growth	To 4' x 1'
Flowers	Yellow and fragrant; open in the evening
Harvest	Leaves, roots, and seeds
Fertilizer	Not particular
Soil	Sandy, medium loamy, well-drained
Tolerance	Drought tolerant
Attracts	Bees, birds (for seeds), hummingbirds (for nectar), and moths
Seaside	Yes
Containers	Yes

USES

CULINARY — Several Native American tribes, including the Cherokee, Iroquois, Ojibwa, and Potawatomi, boiled the roots and ate them like potatoes. The young leaves were cooked and eaten as greens while shoots were eaten raw. A tea was made for use as a dietary stimulant and to treat obesity.

MEDICINAL — A hot poultice, made from the entire plant, was used to treat bruises while the roots were chewed and rubbed into the muscles to improve strength. Evening Primrose has also been used to treat menstrual and bowel pain.

Today syrup is made from the flowers to treat whooping cough. Evening Primrose oil is taken internally for the treatment of eczema, acne, brittle nails, rheumatoid arthritis as well as related liver damage. Regular consumption of the oil helps to reduce blood cholesterol levels and lower blood pressure. The oil is also added to skin preparations and cosmetics. A yellow dye can be made from the flowers, while a finely ground powder, made from the stems, is used cosmetically in face-masks to counteract reddened skin.

MYSTICAL — None known.

GERANIUM, WILD (ALUM, CRANSEBILL)

Geranium maculatum

Family	Geraniaceae – Geranium family
Origin	Eastern North America
Zones	3-8
Type	Herbaceous perennial
Inclination	Non-invasive
Exposure	Full to half-sun
Start	Cuttings. Divisions or seeds
Growth	To 18" x 18"
Flowers	Lavender, pink and lavender
Harvest	Leaves and stems
Fertilizer	Not particular
Soil	Well-drained
Tolerance	Drought tolerant once established
Attracts	Bees and butterflies
Seaside	Yes
Containers	Yes

USES

CULINARY — None known. Flowers of cultivated, scented geraniums can be eaten, but references were not found designating this plants flowers as being consumed by Native Americans.

MEDICINAL — The Meskwaki made a tea from the roots and used it for toothaches, painful nerves and muscles, and the roots for hemorrhoids. Powdered preparations were used to treat open sores and wounds. The Cherokee boiled the root, together with wild grape, to rinse the mouths of children affected with thrush. The Chippewa and Ottawa boiled the entire plant and drank the tea for diarrhea.

Wild Geranium has been used as a mouthwash to tighten gums as well as a styptic to slow bleeding of nicks and cuts.

MYSTICAL — None known.

HONEYSUCKLE (TRUMPET)

Lonicera sempervirens

Family	Caprifoliaceae – Honeysuckle family
Origin	Eastern United States
Zones	5-10
Type	Herbaceous perennial vine; evergreen in warm climates
Inclination	Invasive
Exposure	Full to half-sun
Start	Cuttings or seeds
Growth	Fast to 15' x 15'
Flowers	Red to pinkish-red; fragrant
Harvest	Leaves
Fertilizer	Not particular
Soil	Well-drained, rich in humus preferred
Tolerance	Keep moist
Attracts	Bees, birds, butterflies, and hummingbirds
Seaside	Yes
Containers	No

USES

CULINARY None known.

MEDICINAL Native Americans were said to grind the leaves by chewing them and then applying to bee stings.

Today leaves are dried and smoked for asthma, while a decoction of the leaves can be used for sore throats and coughs.

MYSTICAL None known.

HOPS

Humulus lupulus (H. americanus)

Family	Cannabaceae – Hemp family
Origin	North America
Zones	A2, a3, 1-10, 14-21
Type	Herbaceous perennial vine (technically a "bine")
Inclination	Considered invasive; needs to be trained on a trellis
Exposure	Full to half-sun
Start	Cuttings, (to keep strain true), or seeds
Growth	Fast to 15' x 10'
Flowers	Yellow-green, green, creamy-tan
Harvest	Flowers
Fertilizer	Not particular
Soil	Prefers well-drained but tolerates most soils
Tolerance	Average water
Attracts	Bees and butterflies
Seaside	Yes
Containers	No

USES

CULINARY — None known.

MEDICINAL — The Dakota used a poultice made from the strobilus of Hops as a remedy to relieve pains of the digestive organs, while the Mohegan prepared a sedative from the strobilus and sometimes heated the blossoms and applied them to relieve toothaches.

This species of Hops produces the traditional flavor found in beers around the world.

MYSTICAL — It is said that stuffing some Hops in a bag and placing them under your pillow will help you sleep.

INDIAN PAINTBRUSH (PRARIE FIRE)

Castilleja species

Family	Orobanchaceae – Broomrape family
Origin	Western North and South America
Zones	3-9
Type	Herbaceous perennial – hemiparisitic (such as mistletoe)
Inclination	Invasive
Exposure	Full to half-sun
Start	Divisions or seeds (difficult to start from seeds)
Growth	To 2' x 2'; depends on species
Flowers	Orange, purple, red, yellow, white and combinations thereof
Harvest	Flowers and seeds
Fertilizer	Not particular
Soil	Sandy, serpentine or well-drained
Tolerance	Drought tolerant; do not overwater
Attracts	Bees, birds, and butterflies
Seaside	Yes
Containers	Nos

USES

CULINARY — Various Native American tribes ate the flowers as a condiment along with other fresh greens. Eating too many, however, can cause sickness, and never eat the roots, or leaves, as they are toxic.

MEDICINAL — The Chippewa used a hair wash made from Indian Paint Brush to make their hair glossy and full bodied, as well as a treatment for rheumatism. Nevada tribes were said to use the plant as a treatment for venereal diseases, and to enhance their immune systems. This plant has been alleged to have the same benefits as garlic, but only if eaten in small quantities.

MYSTICAL — Long ago a young warrior tried to paint sunsets with his war paints, but nature's colors were too much for him to match, so he asked the Great Spirit for help. Hearing his prayer, the Great Spirit endowed him with paint brushes that matched the colors he needed. The young warrior then traveled western American, leaving his brushes behind him in the mountain meadows as he traveled, creating Indian Paint Brush plants to grow behind him wherever he went.

LETTUCE, WILD (CANADA LETTUCE)

Lactuca canadensis

Family	Asteraceae – Aster family
Origin	North America
Zones	All
Type	Annual, biennial
Inclination	Reseeds easily
Exposure	Full to half-sun; part shade in hotter climates
Start	Seeds
Growth	To 3' x 2'; depends on species
Flowers	Yellow, yellow-orange
Harvest	Flowers and leaves
Fertilizer	Organic
Soil	Light to medium loamy, well-drained
Tolerance	Keep moist
Attracts	Insects
Seaside	Yes
Containers	Yes

USES

CULINARY   Wild Lettuce plants can be used the same as commercial lettuce. The plants' leaves can be cooked similar to spinach, and the leaves can be dipped in butter and fried like fritters.

MEDICINAL   Wild Lettuce was used by many tribes for sedative purposes, especially for nervous complaints.

MYSTICAL   Older Wild Lettuce leaves contain sedative properties that were often used among Native American tribes in religious rituals. as an aid in seeking meditative trances and visions, and to create more vivid dreams.

LICORICE (WILD), AMERICAN

Glycyrrhiza lepidota

Family	Fabaceae – Pea family
Origin	Western United States
Zones	3-10
Type	Perennial
Inclination	Invasive
Exposure	Sun to half-sun
Start	Seeds
Growth	To 3' x 1'
Flowers	Yellowish-white in dense, long stalks; fragrant
Harvest	Seeds
Fertilizer	Not particular
Soil	Sandy
Water	Medium to moist
Attracts	Bees and butterflies
Seaside	Yes
Containers	Yes

USES

CULINARY — Native Americans ate the roots of Wild Licorice raw or cooked. The Cheyenne and other tribes also ate the tender young shoots.

MEDICINAL — The Blackfoot and Pawnee used Wild Licorice leaves to make a poultice for earaches, while the roots were used for toothaches and fevers. A tea made from the roots was used to speed delivery of the placenta after childbirth, as well as a remedy for coughs, diarrhea, chest pains, stomachaches, and fevers in children.

MYSTICAL — None known.

MILKWEED, COMMON (BUTTERFLY FLOWER)

Asclepias syriaca

Family	Acanthaceae – Milkweed (acanthus) family
Origin	Eastern United States
Zones	3-9
Type	Herbaceous perennial
Inclination	Can be invasive in open, cleared fields
Exposure	Full to half-sun
Start	Cuttings or seeds
Growth	To 5' x 3'
Flowers	Lilac, pink and purple; fragrant
Harvest	Flowers, roots, and seeds
Fertilizer	Not particular
Soil	Sandy loam preferred
Tolerance	Keep moist for best results
Attracts	Beetles, bees, bugs, and butterflies (notably the monarch, of which milkweed is its only source of food)
Seaside	Yes
Containers	Not recommended

USES

CULINARY — Young shoots, flowers and seeds are edible and can be eaten raw or, if prepared correctly, used in soups. The flowers can also be battered and fried, and the shoots can be cooked like asparagus. Flower nectar was used by Native Americans as a sweetener. Caution: In quantities too large Milkweed can be poisonous.

MEDICINAL — Women of some North American tribes used an infusion of the pounded roots to promote temporary sterility.

Today oil from the seeds can be used as a sunscreen. Latex from the plant can be used to treat warts, while various extracts are used to treat asthma, kidney stones and venereal diseases.

MYSTICAL — It is said the Iroquois used the plant to prepare themselves to fight witches.

MULLEIN, COMMON

Verbascum thapsus

Family	Scrophulariaceae – Figwort family
Origin	Africa, Asia, and Europe and has naturalized nationwide
Zones	4-10
Type	Biennial
Inclination	Invasive
Exposure	Full to half-sun
Start	Seeds
Growth	6' x 3'
Flowers	Bright yellow
Harvest	Flowers, roots, or seeds
Fertilizer	Not particular
Soil	Sandy, well-drained and dry
Tolerance	Drought tolerant
Attracts	Insects – both good and bad
Seaside	Yes
Containers	Not recommended

USES

CULINARY — None known.

MEDICINAL — The Cherokee rubbed Mullein leaves in their armpits to treat "prickly rash." Leaf poultices were used to treat bruises, tumors, rheumatic pains, and hemorrhoids. Introduced by European colonists, the Menominee smoked the pulverized, dried root for respiratory problems while the forest Potawatomi, the Mohegan and the Penobscot tribes smoked the dried leaves to relieve asthma, bronchitis, and sore throats. The Catawba used sweetened syrup from the boiled roots which they gave to their children for coughs.

Modern day medicine states that Mullein has many uses. It is efficient in relieving coughs, cramps, allergies, ulcers, respiratory tract infections, as a sleeping aid, a laxative and to get rid of warts. Overall, Mullein provides soothing relieve to lungs and throat.

MYSTICAL — Mullein is said to have the power to drive away evil spirits and to protect one from evil magic. It is worn as a talisman for courage. The leaves are carried in the wilderness to prevent animal attacks and accidents. The plant can also be used in a pillow to guard against nightmares.

OAK, WHITE

Quercus alba

Family	Fagaceae – Beech family
Origin	Eastern North America
Zones	3-9
Type	Deciduous shade tree
Inclination	Non-invasive
Exposure	Full to half-sun
Start	Acorn seeds
Growth	To 85' x 85'; the largest specimen is 144' tall and said to be around 400 years old
Flowers	Inconspicuous, yellow, and red
Harvest	Acorns and bark
Fertilizer	Organic
Soil	Medium loamy to heavy clay
Tolerance	Grows well in dry or moist soils; do not overwater
Attracts	Insects
Seaside	No
Containers	Not recommended

USES

CULINARY   Acorns can be roasted and eaten after leaching the seeds, and the roasted seeds can also be ground and used as a coffee substitute (no caffeine). Native American tribes ground the acorns, after leaching, and used the flour-like substance for a type of bread.

MEDICINAL   Many Native American tribes boiled the bark and drank the liquid in the treatment of bleeding piles and diarrhea, fevers, coughs, colds, consumption, asthma, and a lost voice. The bark has been chewed as a treatment for mouth sores. Externally it is used for skin eruptions, burns, rashes, bruises and as a vaginal douche.

White Oak mulch is said to repel slugs, snails, and grubs. The wood is hard and highly valued for making barrel staves, used for storing wine and liquor, as the wood does not leak. Due to its density the wood is also used for cabinet making, construction, agricultural tools, etc. It is seldom used anymore for medicinal purposes.

MYSTICAL   Oaks are known to attract lightning and were associated with gods of the sky in the ancient world. Carrying an acorn on your person will bring luck and fertility. An ancient Welsh belief is that good health is maintained by rubbing your hands on a piece of oak, on a Midsummer's Day, while keeping silent. The dew under oak trees is a magical beauty aid. Many folks use the wood of oak as their Yule log. Once burned down the ashes are strewn across one's land to bring good fortune, and wealth, in the coming year.

PARTRIDGE BERRY

Mitchella repens

Family	Rubiaceae –Madder family
Origin	Eastern North America
Zones	3-9
Type	Trailing vine - groundcover
Inclination	Non-invasive
Exposure	Dappled sunlight to full shade
Start	Cuttings, divisions, or seeds (seeds are difficult to start)
Growth	To 1' x 4'
Flowers	Small, white; fragrant
Harvest	Berries and leaves
Fertilizer	Organic
Soil	Sandy loam, well-drained
Tolerance	Average water
Attracts	Birds and insects
Seaside	Yes
Containers	Yes

USES

CULINARY Berries are edible. The Iroquois mashed them into cakes, dried the cakes and added water later to make a sauce, or mixed into a type of cornbread. The Mi'kmaq of New Brunswick made a beverage of the Partridgeberry.

MEDICINAL Partridgeberry has a long history as a useful medicine. Native American women used the plant during the final weeks of pregnancy to ease childbirth. A lotion made from the leaves was applied to breasts to relieve soreness from nursing. The plant was also used in abortions and to relieve painful menstruation. The Cherokee prescribed it to stimulate sweating and urination. The Iroquois used it to relieve back pain, vomiting, venereal disease, colic, and children's fevers. They crushed the plant and applied it to bleeding cuts or applied a hot poultice on the chest to reduce fevers.

Modern uses of Partridgeberry include using the berries in jams, pies, etc., and continues to be beneficial in assisting labor in childbirth, as well as relieving menstrual pain and excessive bleeding. It has also been recommended for treating diarrhea and colitis.

MYSTICAL None known.

PENNYROYAL, EASTERN AMERICAN

Hedeoma pulegioides

Family	Lamiaceae – Mint family
Origin	Eastern United States
Zones	5-10
Type	Herbaceous perennial; used primarily as a groundcover
Inclination	Will reseed under proper conditions
Exposure	Full to half-sun; part shade in hotter climates
Start	Cuttings, divisions, or seeds
Growth	To 1' x 1'
Flowers	Light blue and lilac; fragrant
Harvest	Leaves
Fertilizer	Organic
Soil	Sandy to medium loamy, well-drained
Tolerance	Keep moist for best results
Attracts	Bees and butterflies
Seaside	Yes
Containers	Yes

USES

CULINARY — Leaves and flower heads can be used to make a refreshing tea or, in small amounts, as a culinary flavoring. Use caution as too many leaves can be toxic.

MEDICINAL — Native Americans used this herb to treat stomach aches, itching, watery eyes, fevers, and to stimulate menstrual flow. The Onondaga steeped Pennyroyal leaves and drank the tea to alleviate headaches. Today Pennyroyal is also used to eliminate ants and other crawling insects.

MYSTICAL — Pennyroyal in the home is said to end family troubles and help solve menstrual problems.

PENNYROYAL, WESTERN AMERICAN

Monardella odoratissima

Family	Lamiaceae – Mint family
Origin	Western United States
Zones	5-10
Type	Perennial
Inclination	Non-invasive
Exposure	Full to half-sun
Start	Cuttings, divisions, or seeds
Growth	To 2' x 2'
Flowers	Lilac, pale pink, purple and white; fragrant
Harvest	Flowers, leave and stems
Fertilizer	Not particular
Soil	Prefers well-drained, sandy to medium loamy soil
Tolerance	Wet or dry, but prefers moist
Attracts	Bees and butterflies
Seaside	Not recommended
Containers	Yes

USES

CULINARY Leaves can be used to make a refreshing, mint flavored tea, or added to a salad as a garnish.

MEDICINAL The Karuk Native Americans used this plant as a sweat medicine, while women used it as a love plant. The Miwok and Paiute tribes, as well as others, made a decoction of the leaves and stems as a fever reducer, as well as a cure for the common cold. The Paiute and Shoshone also used a decoction to relieve stomach pains and flatulence as well as an eyewash for sore or inflamed eyes.

MYSTICAL None known.

PERSIMMON, AMERICAN (Sugar Plum)

Diospyros virginiana

Family	Ebenaceae – Ebony family
Origin	South eastern United States
Zones	4-9
Type	Deciduous fruit tree
Inclination	Non-invasive
Exposure	Full to half-sun
Start	Cuttings, grafts, or seeds
Growth	To 60' x 40'
Flowers	Whitish-yellow and gold to red-orange; fragrant
Harvest	Fruit
Fertilizer	Organic
Soil	Well-drained, sandy to medium loamy preferred, but will grow in clay
Tolerance	Drought tolerant once established
Attracts	Bees and insects
Seaside	Yes
Containers	Not recommended

USES

CULINARY Once fully ripe the fruit can be eaten raw, cooked, or dried. Native Americans made loaves of bread, and thick soups, by mixing dried Persimmon fruit with cornmeal and acorns.

Today this variety of Persimmon is traditionally eaten in a steamed pudding and, sometimes, its timber is used as a substitute for ebony. American Persimmons are not edible until fully ripened. They are popular in desserts and cuisines. Molasses can be made from the fruit pulp, while a tea can be made with the leaves. The roasted seeds are often used as a coffee substitute. The fruit can be fermented with hops, cornmeal, or wheat bran, and made into a type of beer. Fermented, distilled fruit will make a tasty brandy. As it is extremely hard, the wood is still used to make heads for golf clubs.

MEDICINAL The Catawba Indians stripped the bark from the tree, boiled the strips in water and used the resulting liquid as a mouth rinse for thrush. It was also made into an infusion and used to treat toothaches. The ripe fruit was made into a decoction by Native Americans to treat bloody stools, while a poultice was used externally to treat warts.

MYSTICAL A bezoar (a stone) from the stomach of a goat (who has eaten from a Persimmon tree) is said to be an antidote to poisons.

POKEWEED, AMERICAN

Phytolacca americana

Family	Phytolaccaceae – Pokeweed family
Origin	North America
Zones	4-10
Type	Herbaceous perennial
Inclination	Invasive
Exposure	Full to half-sun
Start	Seeds
Growth	To 8' x 4'
Flowers	Green, produce red berries
Harvest	Berries and leaves
Fertilizer	Organic
Soil	Sandy to medium loamy, or clay
Tolerance	Prefers moist soil
Attracts	Birds
Seaside	Yes
Containers	Yes

USES

CULINARY Because of its poisonous properties the use of any part of Pokeweed for food is not recommended, however, young shoots can be used in salads, and the berries, with the seeds removed, can be used in pies, jellies, etc. The young leaves can be made into a "Poke Salad," but be advised, if used incorrectly, they can be considered poisonous. A red dye is obtained from the fruit and is used as a food coloring.

MEDICINAL The Pamunkey boiled the berries to make a tea for rheumatism, while the Delaware prescribed Pokeweed as a cardiac stimulant. Native Americans in Virginia drank a tea of the boiled berries, while the dried root was used to allay inflammations. Other tribes utilized the plant for arthritis, dysentery, and cancer as well as rheumatism. Berries used in a poultice were applied to sore breasts, while roots made into a poultice were used to alleviate neuralgic pains, bruises, etc.

MYSTICAL It is said that the essence of Pokeweed helps release anger, tension and encourages the flow of energy.

QUEEN ANNE'S LACE (WILD CARROT)

Daucus carota

Family	Apiaceae – Carrot family
Origin	Southwest Asia and Europe; has naturalized in North America
Zones	3-9
Type	Herbaceous biennial
Inclination	Invasive
Exposure	Full to half-sun
Start	Seeds
Growth	To 6' x 3'
Flowers	Light pink turning to white with red centers
Harvest	Flowers, leaves, roots, and seeds
Fertilizer	Organic
Soil	Prefers loamy soil but adapts to most soil conditions
Tolerance	Average water; do not overwater
Attracts	Bees, beetles, wasps and flies
Seaside	Yes
Containers	Yes

USES

CULINARY The young leaves can be cooked as greens, used in salads, or added to stews as seasoning. First year growth of roots taste, and can be eaten, like carrots. The fresh flower heads can be battered and fried like fritters or can be used to make jelly. The seeds can be used to top breads, cookies, etc. Caution: Queen Anne's Lace can be toxic if eaten in large quantities.

MEDICINAL The Mohegan steeped the blossoms in warm water and took the drink for diabetes. Some Native American tribes believed that Queen Anne's Lace increased fertility. In modern times a tea from the roots has been used in the treatment of urinary tract stones. An infusion is used to treat edema and in digestion. A warm-water infusion of the flowers has been used in the treatment of diabetes, while the leaves stimulate the pituitary gland which leads to an increased level of sex hormones.

MYSTICAL The flowers are used in ancient rituals, and spells, for women to increase fertility, and for men to increase potency and sexual desire.

RED RASPBERRY, AMERICAN

Rubus strigosus

Family	Rosaceae – Rose family
Origin	North America
Zones	3-8
Type	Herbaceous, perennial, woody vine
Inclination	Invasive
Exposure	Full to half-sun
Start	Cuttings, root divisions, runners, or seeds (though the seeds may not grow true)
Growth	To 6' x 8'
Flowers	White; fragrant
Harvest	Berries, roots, and seeds
Fertilizer	Organic
Soil	Well-drained and loamy
Tolerance	Average water; drought tolerant once established; does well in moist conditions
Attracts	Bees and butterflies
Seaside	Yes
Containers	No

USES

CULINARY   The fruit was picked and eaten by most North Native American tribes.

MEDICINAL   Red Raspberry has a long tradition of medicinal uses for Native Americans. The Algonquin used the roots for diarrhea, as well as morning sickness in pregnant women. The Cherokee used the roots for coughs and toothaches. A tea was made for menstrual problems, as well as easing pain for women in childbirth. The Chippewa made a tea of the root bark and washed their eyes three times a day for cataracts. They also used the plant to treat dysentery and measles. The Ojibwa used a decoction of the roots for bowel complaints in children. The Iroquois made a tea of the young twigs, while the leaves were used for kidney problems. The root tips were boiled into a concentrated decoction to be used as a blood purifier and to lower, or raise, blood pressure.

Today Red Raspberries can be used to make a blue dye and are grown extensively for the fresh fruit market. Its juices have been used to impart fragrance to soaps, perfumes, etc., while its dried and fresh berries are used in cereals, pies, jams, jellies, etc. The berries contain strong antioxidants that fight against cancer, heart, and circulatory disease as well as age related decline. The oil from Red Raspberry seeds contain a sun protection factor (SPF) of 25-50,

MYSTICAL   None known.

SAGE – ANTELOPE

Erigonum jamesii

Family	Polygonaceae – Buckwheat family
Origin	Southwestern United States
Zones	4-10
Type	Perennial
Inclination	Non-invasive
Exposure	Full sun
Start	Cuttings or seeds
Growth	To 1' x 1 ½'
Flowers	White
Harvest	Leaves, roots, and seeds
Fertilizer	Not particular
Soil	Sandy to medium loamy, well-drained
Tolerance	Drought tolerant
Attracts	Bees and butterflies
Seaside	No
Containers	Yes

USES

CULINARY — None known.

MEDICINAL — Navajo women drank one cup of a decoction of boiled Antelope Sage root during menstruation to prevent conception. A decoction of the whole plant was used to ease the pain of childbirth. The root has been chewed as a cardiac medicine and as a treatment for stomachaches. An infusion of the roots has been used for despondency and as a wash for sore eyes.

MYSTICAL — The Zuni used a leaf of the plant to aid in the treatment of a sore tongue. When done the leaf was removed and, together with a piece of turquoise and white shell beads, was placed in a niche in the river bottom so that it could go to the Abiding Place of the Council of Gods.

SALTBUSH (CATTLE SALTBUSH)

Atriplex canescens

Family	Chenopodiaceae – Goosefoot family
Origin	Southwestern United States
Zones	7-10
Type	Herbaceous perennial
Inclination	Non-invasive
Exposure	Full sun
Start	Seeds
Growth	To 6' x 6'
Flowers	Bright yellow
Harvest	Flowers, leaves, seeds, and twigs
Fertilizer	Not particular
Soil	Sandy and well-drained; tolerates desert conditions and alkaline soils
Tolerance	Drought tolerant
Attracts	Bees, birds, and butterflies
Seaside	Yes
Containers	Not recommended

USES

CULINARY   The Pima ate the seeds, while the leaves were valued for their salt content by many Southwestern Indian tribes

MEDICINAL   The Navajo chewed the stems and placed the pulp-mash on stings caused by ants, bees, and wasps. The Zuni applied the dried roots and flowers, mixed with a little water, to ant stings. A yellow dye can be made from the leaves and twigs.

MYSTICAL   None known.

SARSAPARILLA, WILD

Aralia nudicaulis

Family	Araliaceae – Ginseng family
Origin	North America
Zones	3-9
Type	Herbaceous perennial
Inclination	Invasive
Exposure	Shade to half-sun
Start	Divisions or seeds
Growth	To 1' x 1'
Flowers	Pale green to white
Harvest	Fruit, leaves, and roots
Fertilizer	Organic
Soil	Sandy to loamy or clay
Tolerance	Keep moist
Attracts	Bees
Seaside	Yes
Containers	Yes

USES

CULINARY   The rootstock is used for flavoring in making "root beer." Sarsaparilla was used by Native Americans during wars, and when hunting, for energy and stamina. The roots have a sweet, spicy taste along with a pleasant aroma.

Today young shoots can be cooked as a pot herb. A refreshing tea can be made from the roots and a jelly, as well as wine, can be made from the fruit.

MEDICINAL   The Potawatomi used a poultice to reduce swellings and to help cure infection. Many American tribes used the roots for tea and as a poultice for burns and sores. The Penobscot pulverized dried Sarsaparilla roots and combined them with Sweet Flag root in warm water and used the dark liquid for coughs.

Sarsaparilla encourages sweating for fevers and is stimulating and intoxicating. Used internally it is good for the treatment of pulmonary diseases, asthma, rheumatism, and stomachaches. As an external poultice it can be used to treat sores, burns, itchy skin, ulcers, and various skin problems such as eczema. A drink made from the pulverized roots is used as a cough treatment.

MYSTICAL   None known.

SKUNK CABBAGE, EASTERN US

Symplocarpus foetidus

Family	Aracea – Arum family
Origin	Eastern North America
Zones	3-7
Type	Herbaceous perennial
Inclination	Non-invasive
Exposure	Full to half-sun
Start	Divisions or seeds
Growth	To 2' x 2'
Flowers	Inconspicuous, scarlet
Harvest	Young leaves and roots; can be poisonous if not cooked or handled properly
Fertilizer	Organic
Soil	Bogs and moist places
Tolerance	Always keep moist
Attracts	Flies, mosquitoes, and other insects as pollinators
Seaside	Yes, under swampy conditions
Containers	Yes; best if kept in water-tight containers

USES

CULINARY — Leaves, roots, flowers and young leaves when dried, can be used in soups and stews. The roots can be roasted and ground into a fine powder and added to bread dough or muffin batter, etc. Do not eat any part of this pant unless thoroughly cooked.

MEDICINAL — The Winnebago and Dakota tribes used Skunk Cabbage to stimulate the removal of phlegm in asthma. The rootstock was officially listed in the US Pharmacopoeia from 1820 until 1882 where it was prescribed for respiratory and nervous disorders, as well as rheumatism and dropsy. The plant was also used by Native American tribes as a poultice on splinters and thorns to help heal wounds.

In modern times the rootstock has been used internally in the treatment of respiratory and nervous disorders including asthma, whooping cough, inflammations of the nose and throat, bronchitis, and hay fever. It is occasionally used to treat epilepsy, headaches, vertigo, and rheumatic problems. Externally, it has been used as a poultice to withdraw splinters and thorns from the body, and to help heal wounds. The rootlets have been applied to dental cavities to treat toothaches. A tea made from the root hairs has been used externally to stop bleeding, while the leaf bases have been applied as a wet dressing to bruises.

MYSTICAL — Various Native American tribes wore parts of the plant as a magical talisman.

SKUNK CABBAGE, WESTERN US

Lysichiton americanus

Family	Araceae – Arum family
Origin	American pacific northwest
Zones	6-8
Type	Herbaceous perennial
Inclination	Non-invasive
Exposure	Sun or part shade
Start	Divisions or seeds
Growth	To 5' x 2'
Flowers	Greenish-yellow and yellow
Harvest	Roots and seeds
Fertilizer	Organic
Soil	Loamy, boggy
Tolerance	Keep moist
Attracts	Beetles and flies
Seaside	Yes
Containers	Not recommended

USES

CULINARY The leaves and roots of Western Skunk Cabbage can be eaten if cooked properly. Native Americans ate all parts of the plant when nothing else was available.

MEDICINAL Native Americans used the plant for burns, injuries, sores, and swellings. The roots, made into a tincture, are said to help relieve lung congestion.

MYSTICAL The Cathlamet people of southwest Washington tell this story of why Skunk Cabbage is found near water:

"Before the time of the salmon, Skunk Cabbage was the only thing to eat. When the spring salmon finally arrived, they rewarded the cabbage with an elk robe (the flower) and a club (the stout stalk). As a parting gift the salmon placed the Skunk Cabbage near the music of the river – right along its soft, damp banks, where the soil was best."

STARGRASS (UNICORN ROOT, COLIC ROOT)

Aletris farinosa

Family	Hypoxidaceae – Star Grass family
Origin	Eastern North America
Zones	3-9
Type	Herbaceous perennial
Inclination	Non-invasive
Exposure	Full to half-sun
Start	Divisions or seeds
Growth	To 2'x 1'
Flowers	Small, white, urn shaped on stalks
Harvest	Leaves and roots
Fertilizer	Organic
Soil	Sandy to loamy, moist, or dry, well-drained
Tolerance	Average water
Attracts	Bees and butterflies
Seaside	Yes
Containers	Not recommended

USES

CULINARY None recommended. The roots can be cooked and eaten but leave a bitter, soapy taste in the mouth.

MEDICINAL The Catawba Indians drank a tea of Stargrass leaves for dysentery. The plants were also used by Native Americans in the Carolinas for diarrhea, and an infusion was used as a tonic for general weakness, rheumatism and as a sedative.

The roots are proving to be of great use in treating cases of habitual miscarriage. It promotes the appetite and is used in the treatment of diarrhea, rheumatism, and jaundice. A decoction of the root is a bitter tonic and has been used for treating flatulence along with various uterine disorders as well as dysentery. Large doses of the root can act as a narcotic, a laxative, and may induce vomiting.

MYSTICAL None known.

STONESEED, WESTERN

Lithospermum ruderale

Family	Boraginaceae – Borage, Forget-Me-Not family
Origin	Western North America
Zones	4-10
Type	Perennial
Inclination	Non-invasive
Exposure	Full to half-sun
Start	Cuttings or seeds
Growth	To 18" x 18"
Flowers	Yellow, white
Harvest	Roots and seeds
Fertilizer	All-purpose
Soil	Sandy, loamy or clay; prefers well-drained soil
Tolerance	Drought tolerant
Attracts	Insects
Seaside	Yes
Containers	Yes

USES

CULINARY — Leaves, roots, and flowers can be eaten. Some Native American tribes used the hard, white seeds for food added to salads.

MEDICINAL — The plant was used by the Shoshone and Navajo as a contraceptive. The root was chewed by several Native American tribes as a remedy for colds and diarrhea.

Today the seeds are used for food as well as beads. The roots of Western Stoneseed produce a purple dye which was used by some Western Native American Tribes. A poultice of the dry, powdered leaves and stems has been used to relieve pain in arthritic joints.

MYSTICAL — Roots of some Lithospermum species produce a red dye which was used by Native Americans as body paint. Some people believe this is how Native Americans became known as "Redskins."

SUMAC – SMOOTH UPLAND

Rhus glabra

Family	Anacardiaceae - Cashew family
Origin	Eastern United States with scattered populations in the west
Zones	2-9
Type	Deciduous, perennial small tree
Inclination	Invasive
Exposure	Full to half-sun
Start	Seeds
Growth	To 15' x 10'
Flowers	Yellow, yellow-green, and green
Harvest	Roots and seeds
Fertilizer	Not particular
Soil	Prefers rich, moist, well-drained soil
Tolerance	Average water
Attracts	Bees, birds, and butterflies
Seaside	Yes
Containers	Not recommended

USES

CULINARY   The red berries can be eaten raw or dried, made into a berry tea, and have been used as a lemon substitute. The roots and shoots can be eaten raw when peeled in early spring. Apache children ate the bark as a delicacy.

MEDICINAL   The Omaha boiled the fruits of the tree and applied the liquid as an external wash to stop bleeding. The Natchez used the root of fragrant Sumac to treat boils, while the Ojibwa used a decoction of the Sumac root to stop diarrhea. Various Native American tribes used parts of the Sumac to treat blisters, ulcers, rashes, colds, asthma and tuberculosis, sore throats, as an ear and eye medicine, heart medicine, venereal aid, and for use as a mouthwash and an astringent.

MYSTICAL   None known.

TOBACCO

Nicotiana tabacum

Family	Solanaceae – Nightshade family
Origin	Unknown; believed to be a hybrid of nicotiana sylvestris and nicotiana tomentosiformis
Zones	All; prefers warmer climates
Type	Annual
Inclination	Non-invasive
Exposure	Full sun
Start	Seeds
Growth	To 4' x 2'
Flowers	Yellow to yellow-green
Harvest	Leaves and seeds
Fertilizer	Organic
Soil	Sandy, medium loamy, well-drained to clay
Tolerance	Average water; do not overwater
Attracts	Bees, butterflies, and moths
Seaside	Yes
Containers	Yes

USES

CULINARY — Proteins can be extracted from the leaves which form a tasteless white powder that can be added to cereal grains, vegetable dishes, soft drinks, and other foods, as well as used for whipped egg whites.

MEDICINAL — Native Americans used wet tobacco leaves to relieve bee stings. A decoction of tobacco and herbs was used to heal infected wounds, kill worms, cure boils and rashes, soothe insect and snake bites, cure fevers, hair loss, lung disease, sprains, gynecological complaints, and toothaches. Tobacco also served to still hunger and thirst, and its juice could be used in treating wounds made by poison tipped arrows.

Modern day uses include using juice from the plant as an insect repellent. The leaves can be cleaned and used as an intoxicant as well as externally in the treatment of rheumatic swelling, skin diseases and scorpion stings.

MYSTICAL — Native American tribes regarded the Tobacco plant as a gift from the gods. Tobacco smoke gave Indian medicine men access to higher powers. The water gods were pacified by throwing Tobacco leaves in the direction of the four compass points, while Tobacco was thrown into the water to ensure successful fishing, or into a fire to cast a spell that would protect their tribe from the forces of evil and venomous animals.

WESTERN HEMLOCK

Tsuga heterophylla

Family	Pinaceae – Pine family
Origin	Western North America
Zones	7-10
Type	Evergreen perennial tree
Inclination	Non-invasive
Exposure	Sun or shade
Start	Seeds
Growth	To 230' x 9' (trunk diameter)
Flowers	Cones
Harvest	Needles and seeds
Fertilizer	Organic
Soil	Highly organic
Tolerance	Prefers moist soils
Attracts	Insects
Seaside	Yes
Containers	Not recommended

USES

CULINARY — The cambium layer can be used by scraping slabs of removed bark. The resulting shavings can be eaten immediately, or dried and pressed into cakes for later use. Tender, new needles can be chewed, or made into a tea rich in Vitamin C.

MEDICINAL — A decoction of the pounded bark has been used in the treatment of hemorrhoids, tuberculosis, and syphilis. An infusion of the inner bark, or twigs, is helpful in the treatment of kidney or bladder problems. A poultice of the chewed needles has been used in the treatment of burns. The bark serves as a source of tannin for tanning.

MYSTICAL — Native Americans rubbed their bodies with boughs to ensure hunting and fishing success, and to ward off evil spirits.

WHITE PINE, EASTERN

Pinus strobus

Family	Pinacea – Pine family
Origin	Eastern North America
Zones	3-9
Type	Evergreen, perennial tree
Inclination	Non-invasive
Exposure	Full to half-sun
Start	Seeds
Growth	To 140' x 5' (trunk)
Flowers	Green and yellow-green
Harvest	Needles and seeds
Fertilizer	Organic
Soil	Sandy to clay, well-drained
Tolerance	Prefers cool, humid conditions
Attracts	Bees, birds, and butterflies
Seaside	Yes
Containers	Not recommended

USES

CULINARY The Micmac used the bark to make a beverage, and the Ojibwa used the flowers as food as well as using them in stews.

MEDICINAL The inner bark, young shoots, twigs, pitch, and needles have long been used to treat colds, coughs, flu, fevers, heartburn, headaches, arthritis, neuritis, bronchitis, croup, laryngitis, and kidney problems. Some tribes used the inner bark, or sap, as a poultice for wounds and sores. Pitch was used to draw out boils, splinters, and abscesses, and was also used for treating rheumatism, broken bones, cuts, bruises, and inflammations. A hot resin was sometimes spread on a hot cloth and applied for treating pneumonia, sciatic pain, and sore muscles. This was one of the most important medicines used by the Menominee and other tribes.

Today an extract of the plant has been used in many patented plant medicines for coughs, colds and problems associated with the throat. Many Native American tribes used the pitch from the tree to caulk their boats and canoes.

MYSTICAL A Seneca legend has it that "The kinsmen of the White Pine hold forth the promise of springs' return, and their green robes are the despair of winter and all its furious hosts." ["*First People – The Legends.*"]

WILD ONION (GARLIC)

Allium canadense

Family	Amaryllidaceae – Amaryllis family
Origin	Continental United States
Zones	4-9
Type	Perennial, herbaceous bulb
Inclination	Invasive
Exposure	Full to half-sun
Start	Best from bulbs
Growth	To 1' x 6"; varies
Flowers	White to pink; fragrant
Harvest	All parts of plant
Fertilizer	Organic
Soil	Sandy to loamy, well-drained
Tolerance	Average water; will survive drought conditions
Attracts	Bees, birds, and butterflies
Seaside	Yes
Containers	Not recommended

USES

CULINARY Wild Onion (garlic) bulbs were eaten raw by most Native American tribes. The bulbs were also roasted, boiled, or braised, added to soups and stews, or dried over coals, and stored, for use during the winter months. Wild Onion stalks (leaves) were also a popular food source.

Warning: Wild Onion can be poisonous, to both humans and animals, if consumed in large quantities. Today Wild Onion plants are used as a vegetable, or as a flavoring, for soups and stews among other dishes. The stalks can be added to salads or chopped and used as a flavoring for any vegetable dish.

MEDICINAL The Dakota and Winnebago, among other Native American tribes, rubbed the stalks of Wild Onion over their bodies to protect them from insect, lizard, scorpion, and tarantula bites. Wild Onions help reduce cholesterol, act as a tonic to the digestive system, and help the circulatory system.

MYSTICAL The Monache of California believed the strong odors from Wild Onions were responsible for the Pleiades constellation (six of the stars in this constellation are visible to the naked eye). They believed that the six "Wild Onion women," who were banished by their husbands due to their strong body odor, were these stars. Due to being embarrassed, these six women wove ropes and climbed into the heavens to get away from tribal ridicule. Their lonely husbands attempted to climb after them but were unsuccessful. The constellation Taurus represents their husbands.

WILLOW, NORTH AMERICAN

Salix species

Family	Salicaceae – Willow family
Origin	Worldwide with over 90 recorded species in North America alone
Zones	All
Type	Deciduous groundcover or tree; size varies with species and zone; largest known is Salix nigra
Inclination	Invasive
Exposure	Full to half-sun
Start	Cuttings or seeds
Growth	From 35' to 100' (Salix nigra) largest willow in North America
Flowers	Rose, turning to orange or purple, in catkins
Harvest	Branches, buds, leaves, and roots
Fertilizer	Organic
Soil	Not particular, prefers loamy
Tolerance	Keep moist
Attracts	Ants, bees, butterflies, and wasps
Seaside	Yes
Containers	Not recommended

USES

CULINARY — Boiled, young Willow shoots, buds and leaves are high in Vitamin C. Boiling will make the plant more palatable, but the buds and shoots can be eaten raw if you can stand the taste. Most Indian tribes considered willows as famine food.

MEDICINAL — Due to a chemical from Willow trees that is utilized in aspirin, (Acetylsalicylic acid), willows were highly prized by Native North Americans for their medicinal value. The Cherokee, Creek, Houma, and Seminole utilized a tea for fevers and headaches. The Pomo boiled the inner root bark, and drank strong doses of the tea, to induce sweating in cases of chills and fever. The Natchez prepared their fever remedies from the bark of the red Willow, while the Alabama and Creek utilized willow root baths for the same purpose. Willows were also used to relieve toothaches, mouth sores, stomach problems and diarrhea.

Willow branches are very flexible and are used in construction of basketry, tools, chairs, benches, and fences among other things.

MYSTICAL — Some Native American tribes would lay Willow limbs in the beds of newly married couples in hopes that they would ensure immediate fertility. Others claim that Willows weep because of the losses inflicted on the red man by the white man. Still others say that the Willow trees will stand straight and tall again once an era of peace and kindness among humans becomes a reality. Traditional witches' brooms are said to be bound by Willow branches. Divining rods from willow branches were, and still are, used by mystics to find water.

WITCH HAZEL

Hamamelis virginiana

Family	Hamamelidaceae – Witch Hazel family
Origin	Eastern North America
Zones	3-8
Type	Deciduous shrub or small tree
Inclination	Non-invasive
Exposure	Full to half-sun
Start	Seeds
Growth	To 10' x 5'
Flowers	Yellow to purple or orange-red; fragrant
Harvest	All parts of plant
Fertilizer	Organic
Soil	Moist, loamy, well drained
Tolerance	Average water; do not overwater
Attracts	Bees, butterflies, and insects
Seaside	Yes
Containers	Yes

USES

CULINARY   The nuts (seeds) of Witch Hazel are edible, while a tea can be made from the leaves and twigs.

MEDICINAL   The Iroquois used different parts to treat arthritis, colds, coughs, and dysentery. The Menominee of Wisconsin boiled the leaves and rubbed the liquid on the legs of tribesmen who were participants in sporting games. A decoction of the boiled twigs, used to cure aching backs with steam derived by placing the twigs in water with hot rocks, was a favorite Potawatomi treatment for muscle aches. Witch Hazel was also used by Native Americans as a liniment, eye wash and for hemorrhoids and internal hemorrhaging. The Chippewa used an infusion of the inner bark to treat skin ailments, sore eyes and to induce vomiting. The Mohegan used an infusion of the plant to treat insect bites.

Today Witch Hazel is a component of a variety of commercial health products. It is used externally on sores, bruises, and swellings. It is very useful in fighting acne, psoriasis, eczema, after shave rashes and in-grown toenails. It is also used to treat insect bites, poison ivy, varicose veins, and hemorrhoids. It is recommended to help reduce swelling and wounds resulting from childbirth.

MYSTICAL   The use of twigs as divining rods, to locate underground water, is believed to have influenced the "Witch" part of "Witch Hazel."

YELLOW ROOT

Xanthorhiza simplicissima

Family	Ranuculaceae – Buttercup family
Origin	Eastern and southern North America
Zones	5-8
Type	Deciduous shrub or tall groundcover
Inclination	Root system can be invasive
Exposure	Sun or shade
Start	Cuttings, divisions, or seeds
Growth	To 2' x 6'
Flowers	Assorted bronze, rose, and pink mixed petals
Harvest	Roots
Fertilizer	Organic
Soil	Sandy, loamy, well-drained or clay
Tolerance	Prefers moist conditions
Attracts	Bees and butterflies
Seaside	Yes
Containers	Yes

USES

CULINARY   None known.

MEDICINAL   Native North Americans made a tea for treatment of mouth problems, stomach ulcers and also used it externally for sores, skin conditions and swellings. A tea made from the roots was used by the Catawba and the Cherokee as a stomachache remedy. Today Yellow Root has been found to be healthful in lowering blood pressure and for liver health. The roots have been used to make a yellow dye.

MYSTICAL   None known.

YELLOW SPINE THISTLE

Cirsium ochrocentrum

Family	Asteraceae – Aster family
Origin	Southwestern United States
Zones	Most
Type	Annual, biennial
Inclination	Invasive
Exposure	Full sun
Start	Seeds
Growth	To 3 x 2'
Flowers	Light to dark pink
Harvest	Blossoms, leaves, and roots
Fertilizer	Not particular
Soil	Sandy, medium loamy, well-drained or clay
Tolerance	Average water
Attracts	Bees, birds, butterflies, and insects
Seaside	Yes
Containers	Yes

USES

CULINARY The roots can be cooked and eaten.

MEDICINAL The Kiowa boiled the thistle blossoms and applied the resulting liquid to burns, sores and skin conditions. The Zuni made an infusion of the plant in cold water, let it set overnight and used the liquid to treat syphilis. A decoction of the root was taken by both partners as a contraceptive. Taken five times daily the decoction is used in the treatment of diabetes.

MYSTICAL None known.

Bee Friendly Plants

According to research there is estimated to be close to 20,000 species of bees in the world. More recent investigation shows that this large group of insects is primarily attracted to plants that produce blue, purple, violet, white or yellow flowers. It should also be noted that, despite the above, bees are not usually attracted to plants in the chrysanthemum family, which is the largest flowering plant family in the world. Some popular, common, chrysanthemum species planted worldwide are feverfew, marguerites, Euryops daisies and florist chrysanthemums. As such, if plants from this family are planted around the bee friendly plants listed on the following pages, they can drive bees from your garden. The plants that follow are among the most popular to home gardeners and are not all inclusive, however they should well serve as a beginner's guide to those interested in helping to preserve our planet's fast dwindling supply of bees.

While the decline in bees can be attributed to many factors including pesticides, mites, virus's etc., one of the major players is the loss of native plants due to encroachment by agriculture, and urbanization into habitats that once supported myriads of wildflowers. You can help in no small way by planting one or more of these species each and every year.

SOME HELPFUL HINTS FOR ATTRACTING

A MULTITUDE OF BEES TO YOUR GARDEN ARE:

1. Use local native plants. Research suggests that native plants are four times more attractive to native bees than exotic plants.

2. Choose different colors of flowers.

3. Use flowers of different shapes and sizes. Bees come in different sizes, have different tongue lengths, and will feed on different sizes and shapes of flowers that are suited to their particular characteristics.

4. Plant bee-friendly plants that flower at different times of the year to keep the little guys coming around.

5. Plant flowers in clusters of the same variety to attract more bees. Four feet or more in diameter, per cluster, is recommended.

ANNUALS

Basil	All Varieties
Bidens	Bidens ferulifolia
Blazing Star	Liatris spicata
Borage	Borago officinalis
Calendula	Calendula officinalis
Calliopsis	Coreopsis tinctoria
Centaurea	Dusty Miller, Bachelor's Button, and others – All Varieties, except C. Montana and C. gymnocarpa
Cilantro	Corandrum sativum (also called Coriander)
Clarkia	All Varieties (also called "Farewell to Spring")
Collinsia	Collinsia heterophylla (also called "Chinese Houses")
Cosmos	Cosmos bipinnatus and sulphureus
Cucumbers	All Varieties
Gaillardia	Gaillardia pulchella
Gilia	All Varieties
Lupine	Lupinus densiflorus, hartwegii, nanus and succulentus
Madia	Madia elegans – possibly others – little defined Pacific Coast native
Marigolds	Tagetes erecta (American-African), T. filifolia (Irish lace), T. patula (French) and T. tenuifolia (Signet)
Marjoram	Origanus marjorana - generally treated as a summer annual
Melons	All Varieties
Peppers	All Varieties
Poppies	Papaver commutatum (lady Bird), P. rhoeas (Flanders) and P. somniferum (opium),
Sage	All Varieties

Scabiosa	Pincushion flowers; some are perennials – see "Perennials"
Squash	All Varieties
Sunflower	Helianthus annus (common Sunflower)
Tidy Tips	Layia platyglossa
Toadflax	Linaria "Fantasy Hybrids," L. maroccana and L. reticulata
Zinnia	Zinnia angustifolia, Z. elegans, Z. hageana and Z. peruviana (Many varieties and hybrids – "elegans" is the common variety)

PERENNIALS

Aster	All Varieties, except Aster alpinus
Agastache	Mint Family – All Varieties, except Agastache brevifolia
Barberry	Berberis – All Varieties, except linearifolia and wilsoniae
Bee Balm	Monarda – All Varieties
Blackberries	Includes Marionberry, Ollalieberry, Raspberry, Cascade, Boysenberry, and all other berry producing vines
Blazing Star	Mentzelia laevicaulis
Bluebeard	Caryopteris – All Varieties
Blueberry	All varieties; There are warm climate and cold climate blueberries, so be sure and select those varieties suited to your area
Buckwheat	Eriogonum – all varieties except E. crocatum, E. fasiculatum and E. wrightii
Bush Anemone	Carpenteria
Buttercups	This family is immense and includes Anemone, Aquilegia (Columbine), Clematis, Delphinium, Hellebore and Ranunculus

Buttonbush	Cephlanthus occidentalis
Calamint	Calamintha – All Varieties
Catnip	Nepeta cataria
Ceanothus	Wild lilac – All Varieties, except "Concha" and "Fenderli"
Centaurea	Dusty Miller – C. montana and C. hypoleuca
Clover, white	Trifolium
Coneflower	Echinaceae – All Varieties
Coreopsis	All varieties except C. tinctoria
Cosmos	C. astrosanguineus – "Chocolate cosmos"
Cotoneaster	All Varieties, except C. acutifolius and C. glaucophyllus
Crocus	All Varieties
Currant	Ribes – All Varieties, except R. indecorum, R. malvaceum and R. speciosum, Gooseberries are classified along with Currants in the Ribes Family
Dahlia	All Varieties
Dandelion	All Varieties
Delphinium	All Varieties, except D. cardinale
Fennel	Foeniculum vulgare – All Varieties
Fireweed	Epilobium
Fleabane	Erigeron – All Varieties
Foxglove	Digitalis – All Varieties but some are classified as biennials
Gaillardia	G. aristata and G. grandiflora
Geranium	All Varieties
Germander	Teucrium – All Varieties, except T. majoricum
Globe Thistle	Echinops – All Varieties
Goldenrod	Solidago – All Varieties
Hollyhock	Alcea rosea – All Varieties

Honeysuckle	Lonicera – All Varieties, except L. caerulea edulis and L. hildebrandiana
Horehound	Marrubium vulgare
Horkelia	All Varieties
Huckleberry	Vaccinum – All Varieties; Includes Cranberries and Cowberries
Hyssop	Hyssopus
Hyacinth	Hyacinthus orientalis
Indigo	Indigofera – All Varieties
Lavender	Lavandula – All Varieties, except L. allardii, L. canariensis, L. dentata, L. heterophylla, L. lanata, L. multifida and L. stoechas
Lamb's ears	Stachys byzantina and S. macrantha
Lotus	L. corniculatus - Bird's foot trefoil, Possibly L. scoparius (Deer Weed)
Lupine	Lupinus – L. arboreus, L. argenteus, Russell hybrids and L. Polyphyllus
Mexican- Sunflower	Tithonia rotundifolia
Mint	Mentha – All Varieties
Oregano	Origanum – All Varieties, except O. calcaratum O. dictamnus, O. marjorana, O. onites and O. syriacum
Oregon Grape	Mahonia – All Varieties, except lomarifolium, M. x media, M. nevini and M. trifoliolata
Penstemon	Penstemon barbatus, P. davidsonii, P. digitalis, P. newberry, P. pinifolius and P. rupicola
Perovskia	Russian sage
Poppy	Eschscholzia californica (California poppy, Califoregon poppy)
Privet	Ligustrum – All Varieties
Rhamnus	R. Californica – Coffeeberry

Rhododendron	All Varieties
Rockcress	Arabis – All Varieties
Rosemary	Rosmarinus – All Varieties
Self-Heal	Prunella vulgaris
Small Scabious	Scabiosa columbaria
Spiked Speedwell	Veronica spicata
Sweet Cicely	Myrrhis odorata
Sweet William	Dianthus barbatrus
Teasel	Dipsacus fullonum
Thyme	Thymus sp.
Tickseed	Coreopsis
Toadflax	Linaria vulgaris
Valerian	Valerian officinalis
Verbena	All Varieties, except "Goodingii lilacina"
Viper's Bugloss	Echium vulgare
Vitex	V. agnus-castus – Chaste tree
Wallflower	Erysimum – All Varieties
White Clover	Trifolium repens
Wild Basil	Clinopodium vulgaris
Wild Clematis	Clematis vitalba
Wild Mignonette	Reseda lutea
Wild Privet	Ligustrum vulgare
Yarrow	Achillea – All Varieties
Yellow Archangel	Lamium galebdolan
Yellow Flag Iris	Iris pseudoacorus
Yellow Loosestrife	Lysimachia punctate

TREES

Alder	All Varieties, except A. tenuifolia
Buckeye	Aesculus – All Varieties
Catalpa	All Varieties
Crabapple	Malus – All Varieties
Elderberry	Sambucus - All Varieties, except S. canadensis
Fruit Trees	All Varieties – select for climate and zones
Goldenrain Tree	Koelreuteria paniculata
Hawthorn	Crataegus – All Varieties
Linde	Tilia – All Varieties
Locust	Robinia – All Varieties, except R. ncomexicana
Madrone	Arbutus – A. unedo and A. menziesii
Magnolia	All Varieties
Manzanita	Arctostaphylos – All Varieties, except A. nummularia, A. "Pacific Mist," A. pajaroensis, A. pumila and A. "Sunset"
Maple	Acer – All Varieties
Mountain Ash	Sorbus – All Varieties
Sycamore	Platanus – All Varieties, except P. racemosa wrightii
Poplar	Populus – All Varieties
Redbud	Cercis – Eastern and Western
Tulip Tree	Tulipfera – All Varieties
Willow	Salix – All Varieties

Deer-Resistant Plants

Notice that the title says "Deer-Resistant Plants." Let's be perfectly clear, as far as I know, there are no deer *proof* plants. Like humans, deer will eat about anything when they get hungry enough. When they are little guys, in their first season on Earth, they will sample everything in their path, deciding what plants they like, and don't like. Fortunately, there are plant sprays and numerous devices on the market to keep them out of your garden. Fences for one, electric wire for another, etc. As a rule of thumb, deer do not like plants that give off pungent odors. Indeed, Native Americans would never have had access to many plants edible to humans if deer had not eaten them first. That said, here is a list of plants generally left alone by our furry friends.

Acacia	Bottle Palm	African Corn Lily (Ixia)	Boxwood
African Daisy	Bridal Wreath	Alyssum Saxitale	Buckwheat
American Bittersweet	Bush Anemone	American Sweet Gum	Bush Germander
Ash	Bush Poppy	Australian Bluebell Creeper	Calla Lily
Australian Bush Cherry	Cape Honeysuckle	Australian Mint Bush	Cape Mallow
Autumn Crocus	Cape Plumbago	Basket of Gold	Carob
Bearberry	Carolina Cherry Laurel	Beard Tongue	Carpet Bugle
Beauty Bush	Catmint	Beefwood	Catnip
Belladonna	Cascara Sagrada	Bellflower	Century Plant
Bells of Ireland	Chinese Aralia	Black Locust	Cholla
Blanket Flower	Christmas Holly	Bleeding Heart	Cinquefoil
Blue Bell	Clematis	Blue Fescue	Columbine
Blue Gum	Coneflower	Blue Hibiscus	Crown Pink
Blue Marguerite	Currant	Blue Star Creeper	Cypress

Bottle Brush	Daffodil	Dahlia	Hop Bush
Daphne	Iceland Poppy	Dead Nettle	Ice plant
Delphinium	Iris (most)	Dittany	Ironwood
Douglas Fir	Japanese Barberry	Dracena Palm	Japanese Rose
Dwarf Plumbago	Japanese Spurge	Dwarf Pomegranate	Jerusalem Cherry
English Holly	Jonquil	English Laurel	Juniper
Eucalyptus	Kinnikinnick	Eugenia	Lamb's Ear
Eulalia Grass	Lantana	European Beech	Larkspur
European Fan Palm	Laurustinus	European White Birch	Lavender
Feather Grass	Licorice Plant	Fern leaf Yarrow	Lingonberry
Feverfew	Lilac	Fig	Mauve Clusters
Filbert	Mexican Orange	Fir	Mimosa
Firethorn	Mint	Floss Flower	Mirror Plant
Flowering Quince	Monkey Flower	Forget-Me-Not	Naked Lady
Forsythia	Narcissus	Fortnight Lily	New Zealand Flax
Fountain Grass	Nightshade	Foxglove	Oleander
Giant Reed	Ornamental Fig	Gloriosa Daisy	Oxalis
Gooseberry	Pampas Grass	Gopher Plant	Paper Birch
Hackberry	Peony	Hawthorn	Pepper Tree
Hazelnut	Persimmon	Hemlock	Pincushion Flower
Hispaniola Palmetto	Pine	Honey Bush	Pineapple Guava
Honey Locust	Poinsettia	Ponytail	Sumac
Port Orford Cedar	Sunflower	Prickly Pear	Swan River Daisy
Pride of Madeira	Sweet Hakea	Privet	Tamarisk

Redbud, Western	Tarragon	Red Elderberry	Tea Tree
Red Hot Poker	Thyme	Red Huckleberry	Toyon
Redwood Sorrel	Transvaal Daisy	Rhododendron	True Myrtle
Rock Rose	Verbena	Rosemary	Viburnum
Quince, Flowering	Wandering Jew	Sage (most)	Wattle
St. John's Wort	Salal	Santa Barbara Daisy	Santolina
Sarcococca	Sassafras	Saxifrage	Scented Geranium (most)
Scotch Broom	Sea Lavender	Senna	Shasta Daisy
Skimmia	Snowflake	Snow-in-Summer	Soapbark Tree
Society Garlic	Southernwood	Spanish Broom	Speedwell
Spruce	Squill	Star Jasmine	Statice
Strawflower	Sugarbush		

How To Dry Herbs

There are several ways to dry herbs for future use. One way is to gather your herbs in bunches, tie them with string, or rubber band, and hang them upside down in a dark, well ventilated, and dry room. A small fan directed at the hanging herbs will help them dry faster and avoid mold. Depending on room temperature, size of bunch, etc., it can take anywhere from one to four weeks for them to dry.

A second method is to dry them in an oven. Place a single layer of herbs on a cookie sheet, or something similar (a pizza pan works great) and set your oven on its coolest setting, no hotter than 170°. Turn them over and mix them up every hour or so to ensure even drying. They should be dry within a few hours, or, using a gas oven, you can dry them over a period of days with just the heat from the pilot light. Be careful when using an oven because the herbs can catch on fire if they become too dry. Keep a close eye on them.

A third method is to dry them on racks. You can secure the herbs between sheets of cheesecloth, or window screen, clamp the ends and hang until dry. Be sure air circulates freely between the sheets to prevent mold.

Other ways include sun drying if you live in a relatively moisture free environment (the desert for example), however sun drying has a tendency to bleach the herbs of their potency and is Not Recommended here. Spice mills, dehydrators and food processors also work.

To reiterate, the biggest drawback in drying herbs is the fact that they can readily mold if not dried properly. Keep them out of direct sunlight and keep them in a dark, well ventilated, and dry room (I use a closet leaving the door open with a fan going at least part of the day) to help prevent this malady from destroying your crop.

Once the leaves are dried remove them from their stems, crumble a little bit and store them whole. To make some tea steep 1 1/2 teaspoons of the crushed, dried herbs in a cup of near-boiling water for about five minutes, strain and enjoy. Once again, don't be shy about mixing your herbs. Who knows, you may come up with the world's next best-selling tea concoction!

How To Make Herbal Teas

Why bother growing your own herbs and making teas from them when it's much easier to buy them, already packaged, from the store or online?

Well, making your own herbal tea has many benefits. Among them are inexpensive ways to use your tea for a medicinal drink, or a relatively easy way to just enjoy a tasty beverage, either hot or cold, depending on your mood and the weather. Also, it is well known that using fresh herbs help strengthen the immune system, and detoxify the body, to a greater degree than buying them in a container which may have been sitting around for a long time. Fresh herbs are loaded with vitamins, antioxidants, essential oils, soluble fiber, minerals, enzymes, chlorophyll, and numerous other compounds to boost your health.

To make your own tea start with two tablespoons of fresh crushed leaves, or one tablespoon of your own dried leaves, or seeds. Add one cup of water to a non-metallic pot and bring to a boil. Always use non-metallic cups and pots as metal can taint the flavor of your tea. Add the leaves or seeds and let them steep for about five minutes. Be sure to turn the heat off once the water comes to a boil. Five minutes is an arbitrary time as the longer you let the herbs steep the stronger the tea will be. It's a good idea to cover whatever herbs you are using with a lid to help preserve the flavor of the herb, especially if you are cooking for medicinal purposes, as this will help retain the essence of the herb. Once your newly made tea has reached its desired strength, uncover and strain. After that you can add honey or sugar or lemon juice or whatever you want to suit your taste. For iced tea use three tablespoons of freshly crushed leaves, or two of dried, to help compensate for melting ice. To make two cups of brew double the recipe, etc.

Not all herbs are suitable for teas so make sure the herb you are using is safe, reliable and does what you want it to do. Remember, in most cases, if you can eat an herb, you can drink it. Also, don't be shy. Try different herbs, mixed together, and surprise yourself!

How To Make Herbal Capsules

Many herbs have a bitter, or unpleasant taste, if used in teas, so making your own capsules is a good way to store those you want to use for their medicinal benefits. They are also convenient to take with you wherever you go for later use. Another benefit to making your own capsules is that you know for sure what the contents are. If you buy pre-packaged you have no way of knowing just how pure the herbs are, or how long they have been on the shelf, losing potency over the days, weeks, and months that they sit there. Go fresh! Go safe!

To get started you must first gather and dry them as mentioned on page 249. Use a mortar and pestle, coffee grinder, blender, or whatever, and grind the leaves into a fine powder until you feel you have enough to last awhile.

Next you will need to buy the empty capsules and a capsule machine. These can usually be purchased at your local health food store (or they can order for you – give them a chance and shop locally before you try elsewhere) or over the internet, or possibly at some of the bigger box stores.

If you don't want to use a capsule machine or can't afford one (they are generally reasonably priced and come with instructions on how to use), then you can fill the capsules yourself. First, pack the large end with your powdered herb and then insert the small end. Once inserted, and tightened, shake the powder to more evenly fill the capsule. This takes some practice to get it right so don't give up. Surgical gloves help to keep the dried herbs and capsules from sticking to your fingers if you want to go that route. Use an appropriate storage vessel for your capsules (you can buy these also) and store out of sunlight.

So, now you're all set. It's a pretty good idea to talk to an herbalist about how much to take initially, or go online and see what the stores, and people, there recommend. Or, you can start out taking perhaps a capsule a day to see if they are going to have any adverse effects, eventually increasing the dose to where you think it will be the most beneficial.

How To Make Herbal Oils And Ointments

Essential oils and ointments have many uses both in medicine and aromatherapy. To make your own combine about four ounces of fresh herb (or two ounces dried) with one pint of olive, safflower, or other pure vegetable oil. Heat gently, uncovered, for about one hour. For oil, strain, bottle, and cap tightly when cooled. To make an ointment, add one to one-and-a-half ounces of beeswax to the mixture as it heats. Let cool and bottle appropriately.

When done try a few drops in hot water, or in a facial steamer, to help you relax. Add a few drops of your herbal oil to a spray bottle for an immediate pick-me-up on a hot day, or spray around a room for your own brand of air freshener. After a shower, put a few drops of your special herbal scent on a wet washcloth, rub all over, and air dry yourself. For a great smelling laundry drop 5-8 drops into the wash load. Put several drops in your bath tub to help you relax and refresh your body and soul.

Many herbs make great topical ointments for various ailments, such as rashes, burns, etc. Check the herbs listed in this book for herbs that help relieve these problems.

Understand that herbal oils and ointments on the market are steam distilled and therefore normally stronger than your own preparations, so you need to adjust accordingly. Again, you don't know exactly what they add to the oils on the market, so, to get a true blend of what you want, make it yourself. Another advantage to making your own oils and ointments is that you can make blends of your favorite herbs that you can't find in the markets and amaze yourself and those around you!

How To Make Herbal Sodas

To make your own herbal sodas gather up one-half cup of sugar, three-quarters ounce fresh herbs (your choice), one teaspoon of fresh squeezed lemon, or orange, or grapefruit, etc. Some ice for servings and some sparkling water or club soda.

Pour one cup of water into a medium sized saucepan and cook over medium heat. After bringing to a simmer pour in sugar and stir until dissolved. Remove from heat, add herbs, stir, cover, and let cool.

Pour mixture through a fine sieve and discard herbs. Stir in lemon (or other) citrus juice. Refrigerate at least 30 minutes.

Fill glasses with ice. Add 2-4 tablespoons of your mixture and fill glass with sparkling water or club soda. This recipe makes about 10 glasses of soda. You might want to try cranberry or other types of juices to vary your drinks.

How To Make Herbal Candy

Well, you've come this far, so why not?

First make 3 cups of your favorite herbal tea and make it strong, then gather 3 ½ cups of granulated sugar. Mix together in a large saucepan and make sure the pan is extra-large because the mix will bubble profusely and may overflow. Boil until the mix reaches 292° (see "Altitude Adjustment" below). Next pour into a shallow, buttered pan and let cool. Cut up into pieces before the mix hardens all the way. You can also pull it like taffy for a softer, chewier candy.

Use a candy thermometer to see what temperature water boils at where you live. If you live where the water boils at around 180°, subtract that from 212 (sea level boiling point which is the standard). That comes to 32°, so the boiling point you want is 260°, or 292 minus 32.

There are a thousand and one herbal candy recipes on the internet so check them out for variety.

How To Make Herbal Incense

Okay, now that you've successfully dried your herbs and learned how to make essential oils, let's make some home-grown incense to increase the fragrance of your home, shop, bathroom, dog kennel or whatever.

First, place your herbs into a mortar bowl and crush with a pestle, or use the other methods described on page 249, making sure your herbs are ground into a fine powder. Add wood shavings, such as cedar, sandalwood, pine, or spruce. Most recipes call for a one-to-one ratio, but that will be up to you depending on what scent you are trying to create.

Add some type of resin to hold your shavings and herbs together. Some sites recommend aloe gel, myrrh, amber, mastic or frankincense to name a few. Appropriate resins can be found in many arts and crafts stores or through online holistic stores. Resins keep your incense from separating and help make scents stronger.

Add ten drops of essential oil to your mixture. Essential oils include lavender, juniper, lemon, olive oil and, of course, your own, homemade, much better mix (see "Herbal Oils" - page 252). Essential oils are generally very strong so be careful in how much you add, or you could ruin your brew. Start sparingly and work up to what works best for you.

Mix your powder and oil until fully moist and blended, then cover with plastic wrap and store in a cool, dark, dry room for up to 14 days.

Once your ingredients are dry remove from the drying room. Once done you should be ready to make your own incense sticks, cones or whatever.

How To Make Herbal Candles

While you are at it why not make some herbal candles along with everything else? There are many ways to do this, but the simplest seems to be from an article written by Ellen Dugan for The Llewellyn Journal, which I have altered somewhat.

First you will need to visit your local arts and crafts store to pick up some beeswax sheets (App. 16 x 8 inches), and some wicks, along with a hairdryer if you don't already have one.

If the beeswax you are working with is rolled you will need to flatten it out (gently!). If it appears hard, and may crack when you unroll it, gently warm with the hair dryer, and proceed. Set the hairdryer on low or you may have beeswax icicles hanging from your counter!

Next, lay a piece of wick along the edge (make sure a small piece sticks out the top!) and warm with the hairdryer on its lowest setting. Sprinkle the sheet with your chosen herb (or herbs) and gently press down into the sheet of wax.

Finally, carefully roll up your creation. Your herbs will stay between the sheets as you roll the candle. Once done heat with the hairdryer again. This will mold the edges together and afford you time to set the bottom on a flat surface and gently press, giving your candle a flat bottom to set elsewhere.

Why bother? For one beeswax candles burn longer than paraffin, do not drip, and do not create soot, plus you have the added satisfaction of a job well done, your house will smell great, you can probably sell them if you want, and they make great gifts.

How To Make An Herbal Infusion, Decoction, Paste And/Or Poultice

To make your own herbal infusion (in this case, an extract that results from steeping your herbs) add one tablespoon of dried herbs to one cup of boiling water.

Place herbs in a strong glass container.

Pour boiling water over the herbs.

Cover your glass container tightly so that the steam, which will carry the herbal essence off, does not escape. Do not use metal containers as they can contaminate the infusion.

When the water has cooled to room temperature strain the herbs. The resulting liquid is called an infusion.

Making an Herbal Decoction

To make an herbal decoction, make a stronger beverage. See how easy this book is!

Making an Herbal Paste

What is an herbal paste? Herbal pastes are used to ease the discomfort of sprains, and to help cool painful, swollen joints and muscles. Boils, abscesses, and splinters also have been treated using herbal pastes.

To start, gather a small mixing bowl, two teaspoons (10 ml) of **powdered** oatmeal, four teaspoons of herbal tincture (in this case, the addition of your herbal infusion), clean water, some plastic wrap, and some medicinal tape.

Place the oatmeal and tincture in a bowl and mix together well. If the mixture does not reach the consistency of paste once done, then add a teaspoon of water and keep going until it does.

Apply a thick layer of your paste over the affected area, wrap with plastic wrap and secure with tape. Remove after four hours. You can store your homemade herbal remedy in the refrigerator for up to one week.

Making an Herbal Poultice

Herbal poultices are similar to pastes with some differences. They are primarily used in drawing out infections and to help speed healing. Poultices help by increasing blood flow, relaxing tense muscles, soothing inflamed tissues and draining toxins from an infected area.

To make a dried herb poultice use a mortar and pestle and grind the herb into a powder. Next, place the crushed herb into a bowl and add enough water to make a thick paste. Make enough to cover the affected area.

Spread your herbal poultice over a clean piece of gauze, muslin, linen, or white cotton, then cleanse the affected area with hydrogen peroxide and place the cloth over the wound. Wrap a towel around the cloth and secure with a pin or other fastener. A hot water bottle placed over the cloth will keep it warm and help speed recovery.

To make a fresh herb poultice place two ounces of whole herb (about ½ cup) in a small saucepan, add a cup of water and simmer for two minutes. Do not drain. Pour the mix over the cloth and allow the water to drain. Cleanse the affected area with hydrogen peroxide and wrap and secure the cloth as above. The treatment time will vary from one to twenty-four hours. You will know when the poultice has done its work when the pain subsides. In the case of pastes you apply the herbal mix to the skin and cover, in the case of poultices you apply a paste to the cloth and then cover the skin. Both remedies have been around a long time, work well and are still valid to this day.

There are a multitude of medicinal herbs you can grow yourself that are available in the market place. The best advice I can give is to search the internet, or visit your local library, to find what herbs best suit your needs. A good way to start is to Google "Herbal remedies to help relieve aches and pains", and then set aside a couple of days to search them all.

Aromatherapy

Aromatherapy is a natural and non-invasive way of treating various ailments, including bronchitis, fatigue, migraines, respiratory ailments, acne, arthritis, muscular aches and pains, cystitis, colds, and flu. It also includes assisting the body's natural ability to balance, regulate and heal itself. As herbal essential oils can be used in making incense, breathing in the air around incense can help alleviate cold symptoms, etc., as listed above. More to the point, herbal essential oils are used in massage therapy to help with skin and joint problems, etc., and also leave you smelling pretty darn good! Each separate herb used in aromatherapy has a special aromatic fragrance all its own and, used in massages, is said to relieve stress, among other things. You can also use fragrant, herbal essential oils as perfume, or put a few drops in your bath water for a refreshing bath.

Listed here, in alphabetical order, are some of the more popular herbs used in aromatherapy: Aloe Vera, Basil, Bergamot (Bee Balm), Borage, Caraway, Catnip, Cilantro (Coriander), Clary Sage, Cloves, Comfrey, Cardamom, Dill, Fennel, Feverfew, Frankincense, Hops, Horehound, Hyssop, Lavender, Lemon Balm, Lemon Grass, Marjoram, Myrrh, Orange Mint, Parsley, Peppermint, Rosemary, Sage, Sassafras, Spearmint, Thyme, Valerian and Yarrow.

There are many different varieties of mint on the market, and all can be used in aromatherapy.

For an excellent site on the virtues of aromatherapy, and a more extensive, and informative, list of plants you can use in this practice, visit "Joellessacredgrove.com."

Poisonous Plants

Advice I have given on this subject over the years is simply this:

If you can't buy the plant, or derivative thereof, at the grocery store either fresh, packaged, wrapped, dried, canned, etc., then consider it poisonous. It seems to have worked in the 40 plus years I have been in the plant business. As far as I know, no one has ever died from plant poisoning by heeding this advice.

Also, the people working at your local plant nursery should be able to tell you what plants are poisonous or not.

You're welcome!

Human Ailments and Their Herbal Remedies

Acne	Calendula, Chickweed, Dandelion, Evening Primrose, Feverfew, Lemon Grass, Yarrow
Age Spots	Chives
Abrasions, Scrapes	Calendula, Evening Primrose
Abscesses	Chickweed
Aching Joints	Chervil
Allergies	Chickweed, Evening Primrose, Ginkgo
Athlete's Foot	Calendula, Lemon Grass
Alzheimer's	Ginkgo, Ginseng
Antibacterial	Australian Mint Bush, Bee Balm, Self-Heal
Anti-Inflammatory	Goldenseal, Self-Heal
Antioxidant	Self-Heal
Antiperspirant	Sage
Antiseptic	Bee Balm, Goldenrod, Lavender, Marjoram, Sage, Self-Heal, Thyme
Anxiety	Australian Mint Bush, Bee Balm, Chamomile (German), Lavender (English), Marijuana, St. Johnswort, Valerian
Aphrodisiac	Ginkgo, Mexican Tarragon
Appetite	Bee Balm, Fennel, Lavender, Sage, Summer Savory, French Tarragon, Thyme, Yarrow
Arthritis	Angelica, Chickweed, Evening Primrose, Ginkgo, Marijuana, Marjoram, Oregano, Plantain, Valerian, Violet
Arteriosclerosis	Ginkgo
Asthma	Anise, Chamomile (German), Evening Primrose, Ginkgo, Marijuana, Marjoram, Oregano, Plantain, Valerian, Violet

Astringent	Goldenseal, Sage
Bed Sores	Calendula
Bipolar Disorder	Marijuana
Bites and Stings	Calendula, Chervil, Coneflower, Dandelion, Feverfew, Parsley, Plantain, Self-Heal
Bladder	Garlic, Goldenrod, Lemon Grass, Parsley
Blisters	Chervil, Chives, Garlic, Ginseng, Plantain, Self-Heal
Blood Pressure	Gingko
Blood Circulation	Chervil
Blood Purifier	Bee Balm
Bloating	Plantain
Boils	Chickweed
Bowels	Catnip, Lemon Grass, Plantain
Bronchitis	Anise, Borage, Chickweed, Hyssop, Oregano, Plantain, St. Johnswort, Thyme, Violet
Breath, Shortness	Ginseng
Bruises	Bay Laurel, Calendula, Caraway, Feverfew, Hyssop, St. Johnswort,
Burns	Plantain, Thyme
Calluses	Anise, Hyssop, Calendula, Chives, Coneflower, St. Johnswort, Yarrow
Chicken Pox	Calendula, Dandelion
Chapped lips	Calendula
Cholesterol	Calendula
Circulation	Chives, Evening Primrose
Cirrhosis	Cayenne, Lemon Grass
Colds and Flu	Dandelion, Evening Primrose

Cold Sores	Angelica, Anise, Australian Mint Bush, Bee Balm, Calendula, Catnip, Cayenne, German Chamomile, Garlic, Goldenrod, Lavender, Lemon Grass, Marjoram, Plantain, Rosemary, St. Johnswort, French Tarragon, Violet
Colic	Bee balm, Coneflower, Goldenseal, Hyssop, Sage, French Tarragon
Coughs	Anise, Bee Balm, Caraway, German Chamomile, Dill, Garlic, Mint, Plantain, Savory, Summer, Mexican Tarragon
Congestion	Angelica, Anise, Cherry, Wild, Ginseng, Horehound, Oregano, Parsley, Sage, St. Johnswort, Savory, summer and winter, Violet
Constipation	German Chamomile, Dill (also relieves breast congestion), Ginseng, Horehound, Lemon Grass, Plantain, Sage
Crabs	Basil, Chickweed, Dandelion, Goldenseal, Thyme
Cramps	Savory, winter (intestinal), Valerian
Cuts, Scrapes and Wounds	Hyssop, Lemon Balm, Lemon Grass, Plantain, Sage, Self-Heal, Yarrow
Cystitis	Plantain
Delusions	Valerian
Dementia	Ginkgo
Depression	Borage, German Chamomile, Lavender, Marijuana, St. Johnswort, French Tarragon, Thyme, Valerian
Diabetes	Dandelion, Evening Primrose, Goldenseal, Plantain, Sage, Savory, summer
Diarrhea	Borage, German Chamomile, Lemon Grass, Oregano, Plantain, St. Johnswort, Savory, summer & winter, Self-Heal, Mexican Tarragon, Thyme, Valerian, Yarrow
Digestion	Bee Balm, Caraway, Cayenne, German Chamomile, Chervil, Chicory, Dandelion, Fennel, Feverfew, Goldenrod, Goldenseal, Hops, Lavender, Lemon Grass, Parsley, Rosemary, St. Johnswort, French Tarragon, Yarrow
Diuretic	Lemon Grass, Parsley

Dizziness	Catnip, Marijuana
Ears	Caraway, Garlic, Plantain
E. coli	Goldenseal
Eczema	German Chamomile, Chickweed, Evening Primrose, Plantain, Mexican Tarragon
Energizer	Ginkgo
Emphysema	Plantain
Epilepsy	Marijuana
Exhaustion	Lavender, Valerian
Expectorant	Angelica, Anise, Caraway, Chervil, Hyssop, Plantain, Savory, summer
Eyes	Anise, Calendula, Chervil, Chicory, Coneflower, Goldenseal, Oregano, Plantain, Self-Heal
Fatigue	Dandelion, Goldenrod, St. Johnswort, French Tarragon
Fear	Valerian
Fever	Anise, Bee Balm, Borage, Calendula, Catnip, German Chamomile, Lemon Balm, Lemon Grass, Oregano, Plantain, Sage, Self-Heal, Mexican Tarragon, Yarrow
Feet Sore/Swelling	Feverfew
Flatulence	Mint, Oregano, Parsley, Sage, Savory, summer & winter, Valerian, Yarrow
Fleas	Fennel
Food Poisoning	Self-Heal
Freckles	Chives
Frostbite	Cayenne
Gall Bladder	Lavender
Gallstones	Dandelion
Gastritis	Plantain

Glands, Swollen	Oregano
Goiter	Plantain
Gout	Chicory, Fennel, Parsley, St. Johnswort
Gripe	Caraway
Grouchiness	Lemon Grass
Hangover	Cayenne, Ginkgo, Mexican Tarragon, Violet
Hay Fever	German Chamomile, Marjoram
Headache	German Chamomile, Evening Primrose, Lavender, Lemon Grass, Marjoram, Oregano, Rosemary, Violet
Heart	Ginseng, Self-Heal, Valerian
Hemorrhoids	German Chamomile, Chickweed, Evening Primrose, Plantain, Sage, Yarrow
Hepatitis	Dandelion
Herpes	Coneflower, Hyssop, St. Johnswort, French Tarragon
Hiccups	Fennel, French Tarragon
Hoarseness	Plantain
Hyperactivity	French Tarragon
Hypertension	Yarrow, Valerian
Hysteria	Catnip, Valerian
Immune System	Ginkgo, Hyssop, Self-Heal
Impetigo	Calendula
Impotence	Ginkgo
Indigestion	Angelica, Anise, Caraway, German Chamomile, Dandelion, Dill, Marjoram, Mint, Sage, Savory, summer & winter, Mexican Tarragon, Valerian
Infections	Marijuana, Thyme
Insomnia	Anise, Bay Laurel, Catnip, German Chamomile, Ginseng, Lavender, St. Johnswort, French Tarragon, Valerian, Violet

Jaundice	Chicory, Fennel, Oregano, Parsley
Joints	Chickweed, Mint, Oregano
Kidneys	Fennel, Garlic, Ginseng, Goldenseal, Parsley
Laxative	Thyme
Lice	Chicory, Plantain, Violet
Liver	Parsley, Thyme
Lupus	Fennel, Ginseng, Lavender, Self-Heal, Thyme
Lymph Nodes	Evening Primrose
Macular Degeneration	Coneflower Ginkgo
Malaria	Mexican Tarragon
Memory	Ginseng, Sage
Menstruation	Anise, Calendula, German Chamomile, Chickweed, Evening Primrose, Feverfew, Lemon Balm, Mint, Oregano, Parsley, Rosemary, St. Johnswort, French Tarragon, Yarrow
Migraines	Australian Mint Bush, Feverfew, Lavender, Valerian
Morning Sickness	Catnip
Mother's Milk (to Increase)	Dill, Fennel
Mouthwash	Marjoram, Self-Heal
Muscle Relaxant	German Chamomile
Muscle Spasms	Feverfew, Parsley, Plantain
Muscle Stimulant	Goldenseal
Multiple Sclerosis	Evening Primrose, Ginkgo, Marijuana, Valerian
Nausea	Anise, Fennel, Marijuana, Mint, Savory, winter, Mexican Tarragon, Yarrow
Nerves	Catnip, German Chamomile, Lavender, Marijuana, St. Johnswort, French and Mexican Tarragon, Valerian

Neuralgia	German Chamomile, Lemon Grass
Neuropathy	Ginkgo, Valerian
Night Sweats	Sage
Obesity	Evening Primrose
Rashes	Bay Laurel, Calendula, Coneflower, Dill, Evening Primrose, Plantain, Summer Savory, French Tarragon, Yarrow
Relaxants	Wild Black Cherry
Respiratory Problems	Anise, Australian Mint Bush, Bee Balm, Garlic, Sage
Rheumatism	Bay Laurel, Chicory, Chickweed, Cilantro, Hyssop, Lemon Grass, Marjoram, Plantain, Valerian, Violet, Yarrow
Scabies	Thyme
Sciatica	Lemon Grass, St. Johnswort, Valerian
Scleroderma	Evening Primrose
Scorpion Bites	Mexican Tarragon
Sedative	Lemon Grass, Valerian
Sex Drive	Summer Savory
Shingles	Calendula, Valerian
Sinus	German Chamomile, Marjoram, Plantain
Skin, Dry	Evening Primrose
Skin, Infections	Garlic
Skin, Overall Health	Evening Primrose, Fennel, Thyme
Skin, Sores	Aloe vera, Bay Laurel, Borage, Chervil, Chicory, Chickweed, Coneflower, Dandelion, Dill, Lemon Balm, Lemon Grass, Marjoram, Violet
Sleep Aid	Valerian
Smallpox	Catnip

Snake Bite	Coneflower, Plantain, Yarrow
Sore Throat	Cayenne, Coneflower, Evening Primrose, Goldenrod, Horehound, Hyssop, Sage, Summer & Winter Savory, Self-Heal, Violet
Spasticity	Marijuana
Spleen	Ginseng
Sprains	Bay Laurel, Borage, Lemon Grass, Marjoram
Stamina	Ginseng
Stings	Summer & Winter Savory
Stress	German Chamomile, Ginseng, Rosemary, Lavender, Valerian
Stomach Problems	Anise, Bay Laurel, Calendula, Cilantro, Evening Primrose, Garlic, Goldenseal, Lavender, Marjoram, Mint, Summer Savory, French & Mexican Tarragon, Valerian
Stomach Cramps	Catnip, German Chamomile, Coneflower, Mint, Yarrow
Sunburn	St. Johnswort
Tendonitis	Lemon Grass
Thrush	Calendula
Ticks	Mexican Tarragon
Tinnitus	Ginkgo
Toothaches	Cayenne, German Chamomile, Marjoram, French & Mexican Tarragon, Yarrow
Tonsillitis	Oregano, Violet
Ulcers	Chickweed, Garlic, Plantain, St. Johnswort, Sumac, Valerian, Yellow Root
Urinary Problems	Thyme, Yarrow
Varicose Veins	Calendula, Chickweed, St. Johnswort
Vascular Diseases	Ginkgo
Vein & Artery Protection	Ginkgo

Vertigo	Ginkgo
Vomiting	Basil, Lemon Grass, Marjoram, Mint, Oregano, Plantain
Warts	Chives, Calendula, Dandelion, Thyme
Weariness	Lemon Grass
Whooping Cough	Goldenseal
Worms	Catnip, Garlic, Plantain, French Tarragon
Wounds	Chives, Evening Primrose, Garlic, Goldenseal, Plantain, Valerian
Wrinkles	Chervil
Yeast Infections	Coneflower

Native American Herbal Remedies

Abscesses	White Pine
Analgesic	Buckwheat
Anti-inflammatory	Aspen
Appetite	Boneset
Arthritis	Blue Cohosh – Pokeweed – White Pine – Witch Hazel
Asthma	Dogbane – Milkweed – Oak, White – Skunk Cabbage – Sumac
Athlete's Foot	Bladderpod
Back Pain	Partridge Berry – Witch Hazel
Birth Control	Sage, Antelope
Bleeding – External	Buckwheat – Partridge Berry – Sumac
Blisters	Sumac
High Blood Pressure	Dogbane – Red Raspberry
Blood Spitting	Blackberry
Boils	Stoneseed – Tobacco – White Pine
Bowels	Evening Primrose – Red Raspberry
Breasts, Sore	Pokeweed
Broken Bones	Boneset – White Pine
Bronchitis	Mullein – White Pine
Bruises	Evening Primrose – Milkweed – Oak, white – Pokeweed – White Pine
Burns	Oak, White – Skunk Cabbage – Sarsaparilla – Western Hemlock – Yellow Spine Thistle
Cathartic	Buckwheat

Childbirth	Broom Snakeweed – Blue Cohosh – Partridgeberry – Sage, Antelope
Colds – Coughs	Aspen – Boneset – Broom Snakeweed - Chokecherry – Milkweed – Oak, White – Pennyroyal, Western – Red Raspberry – Sarsaparilla – Stoneseed – Sumac White Pine –Witch Hazel
Colic	Blue Cohosh – Partridge Berry
Congestion	Skunk Cabbage
Consumption	Oak, White
Contraceptive	Dogbane
Croup	White Pine
Cuts	White Pine
Diabetes	Queen Ann's Lace – Yellow Spine Thistle
Diarrhea	Blackberry – Buckwheat – Geranium – Oak, White – Red Raspberry – Star Grass – Stoneseed – Sumac
Despondency	Sage, Antelope
Dizziness	Broom Snakeweed
Douche	Oak, White
Dropsy	Dogbane – Skunk Cabbage
Dysentery	Blackberry – Devil's Claw – Pokeweed – Red Raspberry – Star Grass – Witch Hazel
Ears	Sumac
Epilepsy	Blue Cohosh – Pennyroyal, Western – Witch Hazel
Fertility	Queen Anne's Lace
Fever	Aspen - Boneset – Blue Cohosh – Cherry – Dogbane – Dogwood – Oak, White – Partridge Berry – Pennyroyal, Eastern, White Pine
Fits	Blue Cohosh
Flatulence	Pennyroyal, Western
Gallstones	Blue Cohosh

Headache	Broom Snakeweed – Pennyroyal, Eastern – White Pine
Heart	Buckwheat – Dogbane – Pokeweed – Sage, Antelope – Sumac
Heartburn	White Pine
Hemorrhoids	Geranium
Hiccups	Blue Cohosh
Hysteria	Blue Cohosh
Immune system	Indian Paint Brush
Indigestion	Boneset
Infections	Sarsaparilla
Inflammations	Pokeweed – White Pine
Insect Bites	Broom Snakeweed – Tobacco – Wild Onion & Garlic – Witch Hazel
Insect Repellent	Bladderpod
Kidneys	Dogbane – Red Raspberry – Western Hemlock – White Pine
Laryngitis	White Pine
Malaria	Chokecherry
Measles	Chokecherry
Menstruation	Blue Cohosh - Buckwheat – Evening Primrose – Partridge Berry – Pennyroyal, Eastern – Red Raspberry
Morning Sickness	Red Raspberries
Mouthwash	Sumac – Yellow Root
Muscle Pain	Bladderpod – White Pine – Witch Hazel
Nerves	Geranium – Lettuce, Wild – Skunk Cabbage, Eastern
Neuritis	White Pine
Nursing Soreness	Partridge Berry
Pain – General	Aspen – Boneset – Buckwheat – Dogwood – Geranium

Pneumonia	White Pine
Pyorrhea	Buckwheat
Rashes	Mullein – Tobacco – Sumac
Respiratory	Broom Snakeweed – Milkweed – Skunk Cabbage, Eastern
Rheumatism	Bloodroot – Buckwheat – Devil's Claw – Dogbane – Indian Paint Brush
Milkweed	Pokeweed – Skunk Cabbage, Eastern – Star grass – White Pine
Sciatica	White Pine
Scurvy	Aspen
Sedative	Bladderpod – Chokecherry – Dogbane – Hops – Indian Paint Brush – Star Grass
Skin	Bladderpod – Oak, White – Witch Hazel – Yellow Root – Yellow Spine Thistle
Snake bite	Bladderpod – Tobacco
Sores	Sarsaparilla – Skunk Cabbage, Western – White Pine – Yellow Spine Thistle
Spider Bites	Bladderpod
Sterility	Milkweed
Stings	Honeysuckle – Salt Bush - Tobacco
Stomachaches	Boneset – Buckwheat – Cherry – Chokecherry – Pennyroyal - Sage, Antelope - Yellow Root
Strength	Evening Primrose
Swellings	Bladderpod – Buckwheat – Sarsaparilla – Skunk Cabbage, Western – Yellow Root
Syphilis	Buckwheat – Dogbane – Western Hemlock – Yellow Spine Thistle
Thrush	Geranium – Persimmon
Toothaches	Bladderpod – Geranium – Hops – Persimmon – Red Raspberry – Tobacco

Tuberculosis	Chokecherry – Sumac · Western Hemlock
Tumors	Milkweed
Urinary	Partridge Berry
Venereal disease	Indian Paint Brush – Partridge Berry – Sumac
Warts	Bladderpod
Worms	Chokecherry – Dogbane – Tobacco
Wounds	Broom Snakeweed – Geranium – Skunk Cabbage

ZONE MAP

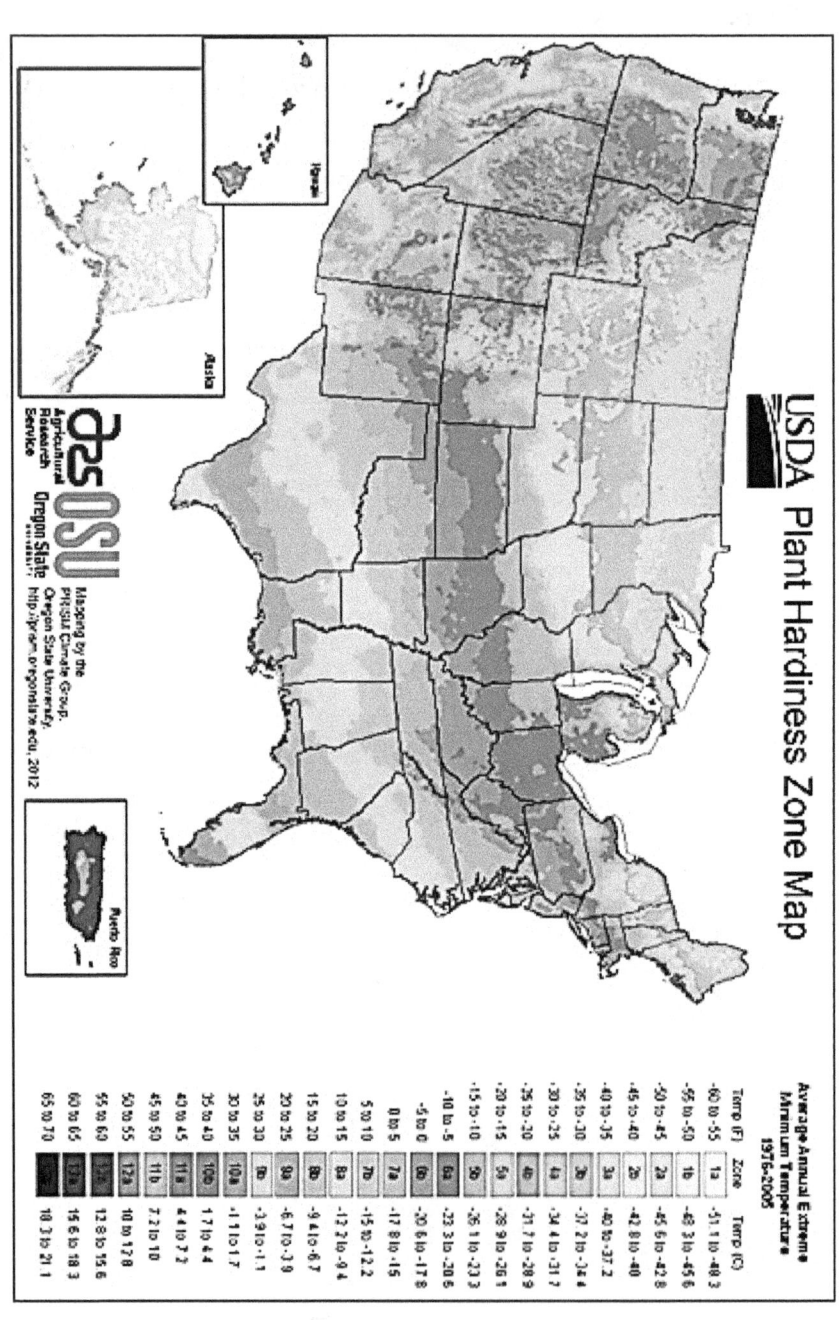

Glossary

ABORTIFACIENT	A drug or device that causes abortion.
ANALGESIC	A drug that produces analgesia; a state of not feeling pain though fully conscious.
ANNUAL	A plant that only lives for one season or less than a year.
ANTIOXIDANT	A substance that slows down oxidation of fats, oils, etc. thus helping to slow deterioration.
ANTISEPTIC	Any substance that inhibits the action of microorganisms.
ANTISPASMODIC	Relieving or preventing spasms.
ASTRINGENT	Contracts body tissues to help prevent secretions, bleeding, etc.
CARMINATIVE	Causing gas to be expelled from the stomach and intestines (to be polite about it).
CATHARTIC	A medicine for stimulating evacuation of the bowels (to be polite about it).
CATKIN	A drooping, deciduous, scaly spike of flowers without petals (poplars, walnuts, birches, etc.).
DECIDUOUS	Shedding leaves on a yearly basis, usually in the fall.
DECOCTION	An extract obtained from herbs by boiling.
DEER RESISTANT	Plants that deer prefer not to eat but may still eat if hungry enough.
DIURETIC	Increases the flow of urine.
DROPSY	An early term for edema.
DYSMENORRHEA	Painful or difficult menstruation.
EDEMA	An abnormal swelling in human cells or tissues – Also a term for the same condition in plants.
EMETIC	A medicine that causes nausea and/or vomiting.

ETHNOBOTANY	The scientific study of plants and their medicinal, religious, and other uses by indigenous peoples.
EXPECTORANT	A medicine that causes or eases the bringing up of phlegm, mucus, etc. from the respiratory tract.
EVERGREEN	A plant that retains its leaves all year as with the conifers – pines, junipers, etc.
HEMI-PARASITIC	An organism that is both parasitic and self-supporting at the same time, such as mistletoe.
HERBACEOUS	Green and leaf-like in appearance and texture.
HERBACEOUS PERENNIAL	A plant that dies back in winter and comes back in spring.
HOMEOPATHY	A belief that the body can cure itself using tiny amounts of natural substances including plants
INFUSION	A liquid extract that results from steeping a substance in water.
OPHTHALMIC	A term that relates to the eyes and their diseases.
PARTURITION	Childbirth.
PERENNIAL	Something that supposedly lasts forever.
POULTICE	Something (herbs) applied to a cloth and then used to cover a sore, rash, etc.
PYORRHEA	An infection of the gums and tooth sockets.
SCIATIC	In the region of, or affecting, the tips of nerves.
SERPENTINE	Something that twists and coils like a snake.
STROBILUS	The cone of a pine, fir, or other conifer – A cone like structure such as the flower of the hop.
STYPTIC	Tending to stop bleeding.
THRUSH	A disease of the mouth, lips, and throat, mostly found in infants
UMBEL	Flower cluster resembling the ribs of an umbrella.

References

American Accreditation HealthCare Commission (A.D.A.M.). "Complementary and Alternative Medicine Guide: Herb, Herb Interaction and Herb Side Effect Links." University of Maryland Medical Center (UMMC). A.D.A.M., Inc., 1997 (Updated: 31 July 2013). <http://umm.edu/health/medical/altmed>

Balch, James F., and Phyllis A. Balch. Prescription for Nutritional Healing, 2nd ed. Garden City Park: Avery Publishing Group, 1997. Print.

Baumgartner, Becki. "Commonly Used Herbology Terms and Definitions." LuminEarth.com: Herbology, 23 July 2010. Herbal Materia Medica, 2010. Web. 2013. <http://www.luminearth.com/2010/07/23/commonly-used-herbology-terms>

Baumgartner, Becki. "How to Dry and Store Herbs – It's Quick, Easy, and Inexpensive!" LuminEarth.com: Herbology, 3 January 2011. Herbal Materia Medica, 2010. Web. 2013. <http://www.luminearth.com/2011/01/03/how-to-dry-and-store-herbs-quick-easy-and-inexpensive>

Baumgartner, Becki. "Homemade Herbal Syrup in Six Easy Steps." LuminEarth.com: Herbology, 24 January 2011. Herbal Materia Medica, 2010. Web. 2013. <http://www.luminearth.com/2011/01/24/homemade-herbal-syrup-in-six-easy-steps>

Bee Guardian Foundation (www.beeguardianfoundation.org/bee-plants)

Benders-Hyde, Elisabeth, Ann Nelson, and David Nelson. "Creosote Bush." Blue Planet Biomes, 19 December 2006 (Modified: 23 September 2010). Brian Schaffner and West Tisbury Elementary School, 2010. Web. 2013. <http://blueplanetbiomes.org/desert_plant_page.htm>

Blais, Pat. "Herb." Gardens Ablaze. Gardensablaze.com, 2001 (Updated: 14 February 2014). Web. 2013-2014. <http://www.gardensablaze.com/Herbs.html>

Blais, Pat. "Recipes." Gardens Ablaze. Gardensablaze.com, 2001 (Updated: 14 February 2014). Web. 2013-2014. <http://www.gardensablaze.com/Recipes.html>

Bogren, Donna. "Myths and Legends About Herbs and Spices." eHow, 1999. Demand Media, 13 September 2009. Web. 2013. <http://www.ehow.com/about_5417655_myths-legends-herbs-spices.html>

Bowman, Barbara. "Arugula." Gourmet Sleuth: The Gourmet Food & Cooking Source, June 2014.

Gourmet Sleuth, Inc., 2000. Web. June 2014. <http://www.gourmetsleuth.com/articles/detail/arugula>

Brenzel, Kathleen Norris. Sunset Western Garden Book. Menlo Park: Sunset Publishing Corporation, 2001. Print.

Burroughs, Jordan Pusateri and Thomas A. Dudck. "'Deer-Resistant Plants for Homeowners." Michigan State University Extension Bulletin E-30421, 2008. Michigan State University Extension – Department of Fisheries and Wildlife, 2008. Web. 2014. <http://www.ipm.msu.edu/uploads/files/deer_resistant_plants.pdf>

Buzzworthy Plants that Attract Bees (www.thedailygreen.com)

Carter, Gary. The Buzz About Our Little Friends, The Bees, Port Orford News, Nov. 3 & 10, 2010.

Chevallier, Andrew. Encyclopedia of Herbal Medicine: The Definitive Home Reference Guide to 550 Key Herbs with All Their Uses as Remedies for Common Ailments. London: Dorling Kindersley, 2000. Print.

"Cooking with Herbs 1-2-3." Mountain Valley Growers, Inc. Mountain Valley Growers, Inc., 1997. Web. 2013. <http://www.mountainvalleygrowers.com/kitchenherbgarden.htm>

Cunningham, Scott. Cunningham's Encyclopedia of Magical Herbs. Woodbury: Llewellyn Worldwide, Ltd., 1985 (2000). Print.

Garden Mastery Tips from Clark County Master Gardner's. "It's Thyme to Try Herbs." Washington State University Extension, May 2002. Washington State University, 1999. Web. 2013. <http://ext100.wsu.edu/clark/wp-content/uploads/sites/7/2014/02/Herbs.pdf>

"Edible Plants." Montana Plant Life. Montana Plant Life, 2003. Web. 2013. <montana.plant-life.org>

Gaylord, Susan, and Jeanine M. Davis. "Glossary of Herbal Terms. "North Carolina Consortium on Natural Medicines, 29 December 2011. North Carolina State University and University of North Carolina, 6 June 2013 (Updated: 18 September 2014). Web. 2013. <http://naturalmedicinesofnc.org/glossary.html>

"Herbal Medicines & Teas." Manataka American Indian Council. Manataka American Indian Council, 1997. Web. 2013. <http://manataka.org/herbalmedicines.html>

"How the Medicinal Herbs Heal." Natural Medicinal Herbs. Spiritual-Knowledge and Led Ziarovky, 1999. Web. 2013. <http://www.naturalmedicinalherbs.net/herbs/medicinal>

Jeanroy, Amy. "How to Brew All Types of Herb Teas: Brewing All Type of Herb Tea Mixtures." About Home, 2008. About, Inc., 1 May 1997 (Updated: 22 February 2012; 11 November 2014). Web. 2014. <http://herbgardens.about.com/od/culinary/a/How-To-Brew-All-Types-Of-Herb-Tea.htm>

Jeanroy, Amy. "Types of Herbs: Medicinal Herbs, Culinary Herbs and Ornamental Herbs." About Home, April 2014. About, Inc., 1 May 1997 (Updated: 22 February 2012 and 11 November 2014). Web. 2014. <http://herbgardens.about.com/od/herbbasics/u/HerbProfiles.htm>

Keoke, Emory Dean and Mary Kay Porterfield. American Indian Contributions to the World. New York: Chelsea House, 2005. Print.

Marie, Sandy. "Drying Herbs: Three Methods to Yield High Quality." Herbal How To Guide. Sandy Marie and Herbal How To Guide, 17 February 2009 (11 December 2009; 12 March 2011). Web. 2013-2014. <http://www.herbal-howto-guide.com/drying-herbs.html>

Marie, Sandy. "Herbal Tea: Making an Awesome Cup of Tea – Every Time!" Herbal How To Guide. Sandy Marie and Herbal How To Guide, 17 February 2009 (11 December 2009; 12 March 2011). Web. 2013-2014. <http://www.herbal-howto-guide.com/herbal-tea.html>

Marie, Sandy. "Making a Decoction, Simple Steps." Herbal How To Guide. Sandy Marie and Herbal How To Guide, 17 February 2009 (11 December 2009; 12 March 2011). Web. 2013-2014. <http://www.herbal-howto-guide.com/decoction.html>

Marie, Sandy. "Making an Herbal Infusion is Easy." Herbal How To Guide. Sandy Marie and Herbal How To Guide, 17 February 2009 (11 December 2009; 12 March 2011). Web. 2013-2014. <http://www.herbal-howto-guide.com/infusion.html>

Mayo Clinic Staff. "Herbal Supplements May Not Mix with Heart Medicines." Mayo Clinic, 10 October 2014. Mayo Foundation for Medical Education and Research, 1998. Web. 2014. <http://www.mayoclinic.org/healthy-living/consumer-health/in-depth/herbal-supplements/art-20046488>

McClafferty, Casey. "Medical Attributes of Hamamelis virginiana – Witch Hazel." Wilkes University, July 2003. Kenneth M. Klemow and Wilkes University Biology Department, 9 April 2001. Web. March 2014. <http://klemow.wilkes.edu/Hamamelis.html>

"Medicinal Plants." Montana Plant Life. Montana Plant Life, 2003. Web. 2013. <montana.plant-life.org>

Mihesuah, Devon Abbott. "Medicinal Plant Used by the Five Tribes in Indian Territory." AIHDP/American Indian Health and Diet Project, 1999. University of Nebraska Press, 2005. Web. 2013. <http://www.aihd.ku.edu/health/MedicinalPlantsoftheFiveTribes.html>

Mindell, Earl. Herb Bible. New York: Simon & Schuster/Fireside, 1992. Print.

Moerman, Dan. "Native American Ethnobotany: A Database of Foods, Drugs, Dyes and Fibers of Native American Peoples, Derived from Plants." University of Michigan Library – Archaeology Reference Books, 14 May 2003. Portland: Timber Press, 1998. Web. 2013. <http://herb.umd.umich.edu>

Mohammed, Gina. "Ask the Doctor: Herbs for Headaches." Mother Earth Living: Healthy Homes, Natural Health, Green Living, June/July 2012. Ogden Publications, Inc., 1999. Web. 2013. <http://www.motherearthliving.com/health-and-wellness/herbs-for-headaches-zm0z12jjzdeb.aspx>

Native Plants of the Northwest, Wallace W. Hansen Nursery (www.nwplants.com)

"Natural Remedies Adult Ailments List." Manataka American Indian Council. Manataka American Indian Council, 1997. Web. 2013. <http://www.manataka.org/page893.html>

Needham, William. "Bee Balm." Hiker's Notebook. William Needham, 24 May 2013. Web. 2013. <http://hikersnotebook.net/Bee+Balm>

Needham, William. "Chicory." Hiker's Notebook. William Needham, 24 May 2013. Web. 2013. <http://hikersnotebook.net/Chicory>

Needham, William. "Coneflower." Hiker's Notebook. William Needham, 24 May 2013. Web. 2013. <http://hikersnotebook.net/Black-eyed+Susan+and+Green+Black+Coneflower>

Needham, William. "Dandelion." Hiker's Notebook. William Needham, 24 May 2013. Web. 2013. <http://hikersnotebook.net/Dandelion>

Needham, William. "Goldenrod." Hiker's Notebook. William Needham, 24 May 2013. Web. 2013. <http://hikersnotebook.net/Goldenrod>

Needham, William. Mullein." Hiker's Notebook. William Needham, 24 May 2013. Web. 2013. <http://hikersnotebook.net/Mullein>

Needham, William. "Violet." Hiker's Notebook. William Needham, 24 May 2013. Web. 2013. <http://hikersnotebook.net/Violet>

Nolan, Judy. "Native American Herbal Remedies." Healing with Nature. Judy Nolan, n.d. Web.2013. <http://judynolan-ivil.tripod.com/id28.html>

"Organic Dried Herbs." Richters Herbs, 1997. Otto Richter and Sons Limited, 1997. Web. 2013. <https://www.richters.com>

Orzolek, Michael, and Keppy Arnoldsen, Aimée Voisin and Jen Johnson. "Herbs Directory: Anise, Hyssop and Marjoram." Pennsylvania State Extension, 1999. Pennsylvania State University – College of Agricultural Sciences, 1999. Web. February 2013.http://extension.psu.edu/plants/gardening/herbs

Pacific Northwest Plants for Native Bees (www.xerces.org)

Pacific Northwest Flowering Shrubs (www.OregonState.edu)

Persson, Barbara. "Annuals, Perennials and Biennial Herbs in Your Garden." Washington State University Kittitas County Extension, 19 February 2014. Washington State University, 1999. Web. 2014. <http://ext100.wsu.edu/kittitas/wpcontent/uploads/sites/19/2014/02/

Annual-Perennial-and-Biennial-Herbs-in-Your-Garden1.pdf>

Pietlukiewicz, Kerry. "Medical Attributes of Hydrastis canadensis – Goldenseal." Wilkes University, July 1999. Kenneth M. Klemow and Wilkes University Biology Department, 9 April 2001. Web. March 2014. <http://klemow.wilkes.edu/Hydrastis.html

"Plant Files: The Largest Plant Identification Reference Guide – Dave's Garden." Dave's Garden, 2000. Lifestyle Home & Gardens – An Internet Brands, Inc. Property, 2000. Web. 2012. <http://davesgarden.com/guides/pt>

"Poisonous Plants." Montana Plant Life. Montana Plant Life, 2003. Web. 2013. <montana.plant-life.org>

"Preparing Garden Soil." Garden Soil. NA MEDIA, 2001. Web. 2012. <http://www.gardensoil.com>

Prindle, Tara. "Food & Recipes." Native Tech: American Technology and Art, 2013. Native Web, 1994. Web. 2013. <http://www.nativetech.org>

Purdue University Administrator. "Herbal Remedies Info." Horticulture & Landscape Architecture. Purdue University, 2010. Web. 2013. <www.herbalremediesinfo.com/HERBS.html>

Robinson, Georgina, and George Agurkis, Anthony Scerbo. "Medical Attributes of Eupatorium perfotiatum – Boneset." Wilkes University, July 2007. Kenneth M. Klemow and Wilkes University Biology Department, 9 April 2001. Web. March 2014. <http://klemow.wilkes.edu/Eupatorium.html>

Rosenbloom, Perry. "Montana Fish and Wildlife." Glacier National Park Travel Guide. Perry Rosenbloom, 2008. Web. 2013. <http://www.glacier-national-park-travel-guide.com>

Stuart, Malcolm. The Encyclopedia of Herbs and Herbalism. Woodbury: Llewellyn Worldwide Ltd., 2013. Print.

The American Association of Naturopathic Physicians. Nature's Pharmacy: Your Guide to Healing Foods, Herbs, Supplement & Homeopathic Remedies. Lincolnwood: Publications International, Ltd., 2001. Print.

UBG Seasonal Recommended Plant Lists. (www.nature.berkeley.edu/urbanbeegardens/list.html)

Wahl, Kirk. "Medicinal Herbal Actions List." Living Afield, 2011. Living Afield, 2011. Web. 2013. <http://livingafield.com/Documents/Medicinal%20Herbal%20Actions%20List.doc>

Wahl, Kirk. "Michigan Medicinal Wild Plant and Identification and Use." Living Afield, 2014. Living Afield, 2011. Web. 2013. <http://www.livingafield.com/Plants_Medicinal.htm>

Weed, Susun S. "Herbalism." Weed Wanderings Newsletter – Herbal Medicine with Susun Weed, January 2003: Vol. 3, No. 1. Susun Weed, 30 March 2001. Web. 2013. <http://www.susunweed.com/Weed_letter_Jan03.htm#wisewoman>

Weed, Susun S. "Menopausal Years – The Wise Woman Way." The Wise Woman Web, 2000. Susun Weed, 30 March 2001. Web. 2013. <http://www.wisewomanwe.com>

Weed, Susun S. "HERBAL PHARMACY: Picking and Drying Herbs." Wise Woman Herbal Ezine with Susun Weed, April 2007: Vol. 7, No. 4. Susun Weed, 30 March 2001. Web. 2013. <http://www.susunweed.com/herbal_ezine/April07/wisewoman.htm>

"Wild Herbs." United States Forest Service. United States Forest Service, 2000. Web. 2012-2013. <http://www.fs.fed.us>

Woodward, Penny. "Herbs and Spices." Encyclopedia of Food and Culture, 2003. Encyclopedia.com, 2014. Web. 2013. <http://www.encyclopedia.com/topic/Herbs_and_Spices.aspx>

About the Author

Gary Carter was born in San Diego, California in 1938 and graduated from Sweetwater Union High School (National City, CA) in June of 1956. After serving three years in the United States Marine Corps he attended college as a science major at Grossmont Community College, continuing his education at San Diego State University as a Botany major. His poems have appeared in the Port Orford News as well as the Las Vegas Sun and many poetry journals and magazines. He is the author of *Jump Start,* an apocalyptic science fiction thriller (2003), *For the Good of the Many,* a National Award winning military/political thriller (2007), *Mystic Summer,* a multi-cultural love story (2010), *My City by the Sea,* Poems for All Ages (2006), *Imagery,* Poems to Make You Laugh, Cry, Wonder, Doubt and Argue About (2013). *The Cedars of Lebanon,* a science fiction, time travel thriller (2018), and "*Songs from the Southern Oregon Coast*", a compilation of short stories and poems, by 56 authors, telling what they love about living along the Southern Oregon Coast, one of the world's most beautiful places. Gary lives in Port Orford, Oregon, where he operates a small nursery in the summer and works on his writing in the winter. He is the father of four, the grandfather of 13 and the great-grandfather of 14.

Also By Gary Carter

Jump Start (2003). Where will you hide when the invasion begins? *Jump Start* is an apocalyptic science fiction thriller, providing an alternate truth to the myths surrounding dragons, UFO's, alien abductions, and all the rest.

ISBN: 1-4137-0194-0

For the Good of the Many (2007). A military-political thriller: With the world on the brink of war over dwindling oil supplies, one man holds the key to world peace but, will he live to unlock the door? In 2007 this novel was presented the Silver Star Award by the Military Writers Society of America (MWSA) for excellence in military fiction.

ISBN: 1-4241-3851-5

Mystic Summer (2008). When young Scott James meets a beautiful Mexican maiden by the name of Henrietta Herrara, from the opposite side of the tracks, the troubles and sparks begin to fly. Journey back to 1954 when it was the greatest time in American history to be a teenager. Or was it?

"Stunning in its presentation," as reported by reviewer Tobe Porter.

ISBN: 978-1-4489-4876-5

My City by the Sea (2006). This short book has poems for all ages and includes four award winning poems.

Imagery (2013). Poems to make you Laugh, Cry, Wonder, Doubt and Argue About.

All books (except *My City by the Sea*) can be ordered at any bookstore, brick, and mortar, online, or from Gary Carter directly. He can be contacted at gcarter123@frontier.com and welcomes your comments or criticisms.

NEW ON THE MARKET

The Cedars of Lebanon (2018). Travel back in time to ancient Phoenicia where three women on a mission to save planet Earth, after a devastating war in the Mideast, are sent to collect seeds, saplings, and cuttings in an effort to propagate them and restore the Levant to its original beauty. But the girls don't return as scheduled and a rescue mission, to try and bring them back dead or alive, is sent back, but things don't go as planned. Will the mission to save the girls, and our planet, fail, or will it be a success?

Songs From The Southern Oregon Coast (2018). Poems and short stories from 56 writers living on the southern Oregon coast. With each poem and story layers of history, culture and inspiration reveal themselves. From the pristine natural settings to the vibrant town atmospheres the region comes to life in this collection.

About the Press

Unsolicited Press is a small press in Portland, Oregon. The team produces fiction, poetry, and nonfiction. Learn more at www.unsolicitedpress.com.

www.ingramcontent.com/pod-product-compliance
Lightning Source LLC
Chambersburg PA
CBHW080214040426
42333CB00044B/2657